THE
PEDIATRIC
ABACUS

THE
PEDIATRIC
ABACUS

Melvin L. Cohen, MD, FAAP
Director, Department of Medical Education
Phoenix Children's Hospital, Phoenix, Arizona

David Rifkind, MD, PhD, FACP
Formerly Professor, Department of Medicine
College of Medicine, University of Arizona, Tucson, Arizona

The Parthenon Publishing Group
International Publishers in Medicine, Science & Technology

A CRC PRESS COMPANY
BOCA RATON   LONDON   NEW YORK   WASHINGTON, D.C.

Library of Congress Cataloging-in-Publication Data
Cohen, Melvin L.
    The pediatric abacus : review of clinical formulas and how to use them /
Melvin L. Cohen, David Rifkind.
        p. ; cm.
    Includes bibliographic references and index.
    ISBN 1-84214-147-3 (alk. paper)
    1. Pediatrics—Formulae, receipts, prescriptions—Handbooks, manuals, etc.
2. Clinical medicine—Mathematics—Handbooks, manuals, etc.
3. Reference values (Medicine)—Handbooks, manuals, etc. I. Rifkind, David.
II. Rifkind, David. Medical abacus. III. Title.
    [DNLM: 1. Diagnostic Techniques and Procedures—Child—Handbooks.
2. Mathematics—Handbooks. 3. Reference
Values—Child—Handbooks. WS 39 C678p 2002]
RJ560 .C62 2002
618.92′0002′12—dc21   2002022050

British Library Cataloguing-in-Publication Data
Cohen, Melvin L.
    The pediatric abacus: review of clinical formulas and how to use them
    1. Pediatrics – Handbooks, manuals, etc. 2. Clinical medicine – Mathematics –
    Formulae – Handbooks, manuals, etc.
    I. Title II. Rifkind, David
    618.9′2′000212
    ISBN 1-84214-147-3

Published in the USA by
The Parthenon Publishing Group
345 Park Avenue South, 10th Floor
New York, NY 10010, USA

Published in the UK and Europe by
The Parthenon Publishing Group
23–25 Blades Court, Deodar Road
London, SW15 2NU, UK

Typeset by Siva Math Setters, Chennai, India
Printed and bound by J.W. Arrowsmith Ltd., Bristol, UK

CONTENTS

CARDIOVASCULAR SYSTEM

ELECTROLYTES AND WATER

Contents

RENAL FUNCTION

STATISTICS

PREFACE

The Pediatric Abacus was compiled in recognition of the fundamental theorem of pediatrics, that children are not simply small adults. It brings together in a single readily accessible volume the basic mathematical formulas that are useful in pediatric practice.

This book is an extensively revised and augmented derivative of *The Medical Abacus*. Formulas and illustrative materials uniquely relevant to pediatrics were added. Formulas relevant to all age groups were supplemented with age-related standards where appropriate, and those of use only in adult medicine were deleted. This work is thus uniquely applicable to pediatricians and those other physicians whose patients include the younger age groups.

It is suggested that an electronic calculator be used with these formulas to minimize the chance of arithmetic errors. Any laboratory results given in SI units are to be converted to conventional units before use (see appendix B). Finally, the results and interpretations should be evaluated for plausibility in light of the patient's clinical status and course.

The authors gratefully acknowledge the counsel and assistance of the publisher's editorial staff.

Melvin L. Cohen and David S. Rifkind
March 2002

ACID–BASE BALANCE

HENDERSON–HASSELBALCH EQUATION

Use

To calculate pH of blood from the arterial bicarbonate concentration (HCO_3) and the arterial CO_2 tension ($PaCO_2$). While arterial blood provides the standard, arterialized capillary blood in infants and children is an acceptable alternative for pH, $PaCO_2$ and HCO_3.

Formula

$$pH = 6.1 + \log\left(\frac{HCO_3}{0.03 \times PaCO_2}\right)$$

pH	=	arterial pH
HCO_3	=	arterial bicarbonate (mEq/l)
$PaCO_2$	=	arterial CO_2 tension (mmHg)

Interpretation

Pediatric normal values

Age	pH	SD	$PaCO_2$ (mmHg)	SD	HCO_3 mEq/l	SD	Sample
Preterm (1 week)	7.34	0.06	31	3	17.2	1.2	arterialized capillary
Preterm (6 weeks)	7.38	0.02	35	6	21.9	4.4	arterialized capillary
Term (birth)	7.24	0.05	49	10	20.0	2.8	umbilical artery
Term (1 h)	7.37	0.05	34	9	19.0	2.3	umbilical artery
3–6 months	7.39	0.03	36	3	22.0	1.9	arterialized capillary
21–24 months	7.40	0.02	35	3	21.8	1.6	arterialized capillary
3.5–5.4 years	7.39	0.04	37	4	22.5	1.3	artery
5.5–12 years	7.40	0.03	38	3	23.1	1.2	artery
12.5–17.4 years	7.38	0.03	41	3	24.0	1.0	artery
Adult males	7.39	0.01	41	2	25.2	1.0	artery

For practical purposes, pH should be at the normal adult value soon after the newborn period. HCO_3, however, is near 20 mEq/l at birth and gradually rises to adult levels (25 mEq/l) in adolescence. $PaCO_2$ likewise begins near 35 mmHg after the newborn period and gradually rises to 40 mmHg. The proportionately low values of HCO_3 and $PaCO_2$ in infants and children maintain pH near 7.40 throughout childhood.

The arterial bicarbonate concentration is maintained by renal function (metabolic), and the arterial CO_2 tension is maintained by pulmonary function (respiratory). When one factor deviates, the other tends to move in the same direction in order to maintain the normal HCO_3/CO_2 ratio and thereby preserve a normal pH. In general, during an acid–base imbalance due to a single disturbance (simple imbalance), the pH is not returned completely to normal. Accordingly, when there is a disturbance, as evidenced by abnormal levels of HCO_3 or $PaCO_2$ with a normal pH, this suggests that more than one acid–base imbalance is occurring simultaneously (mixed imbalance).

References

Cogan MG. *Fluid and Electrolyte Physiology and Pathophysiology*. Norwalk, CT: Appleton & Lange, 1991:176

Effros RM, Widell JL. Acid–base balance. In Murray JF, Nadel JA, eds. *Textbook of Respiratory Medicine*, 2nd edn. Philadelphia, PA: WB Saunders, 1994:175–98

Schwartz GJ. General principles of acid–base physiology. In Holliday MA, Barratt TM, Avner ED, eds. *Pediatric Nephrology*, 3rd edn. Baltimore, MD: Williams & Wilkins, 1994:235

ACID–BASE MAP

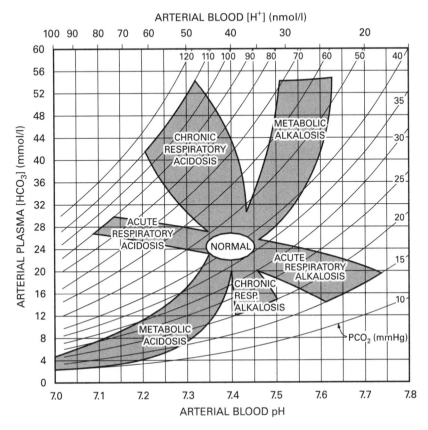

Reproduced with permission from Bremner B, Coe FL, Rector FC Jr. *Renal Physiology in Health and Disease*. Philadelphia, PA: WB Saunders, 1987:12

SIMPLE ACID–BASE IMBALANCE

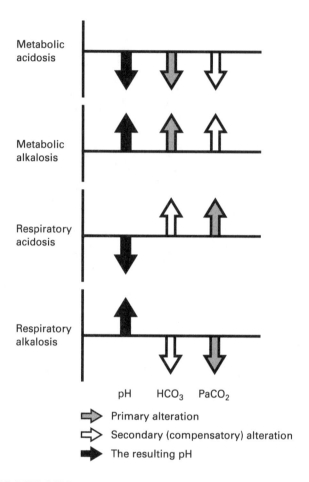

METABOLIC ACIDOSIS

Use

To identify the expected respiratory compensation in metabolic acidosis, and to determine whether the imbalance exists alone (simple) or is accompanied by one or more additional acid–base disturbances (mixed). In acute states of metabolic acidosis, maximal respiratory compensation occurs quickly, and the $PaCO_2$ will reach expected levels in 4–6 hours. For practical purposes, therefore, $PaCO_2$ should be considered a reflection of a steady state (acute *or* chronic state) of a simple or mixed disturbance.

Definition

> pH < 7.35
> HCO_3 more than 3.0 mEq/l below normal for age

Formulas for respiratory compensation

Adult: Expected $PaCO_2 = (1.5 \times HCO_3) + 8$

or

Adult: Expected $PaCO_2 = 40 - [1.25 \times (25 - AB)]$

Child: Expected $PaCO_2 = NPaCO_2 - [1.25 \times (NB - AB)]$

$PaCO_2$	=	arterial CO_2 tension (mmHg)
$NPaCO_2$	=	normal $PaCO_2$ in infants and children (mmHg) – see Henderson–Hasselbalch equation
NB	=	normal bicarbonate in infants and children (mEq/l) – see Henderson–Hasselbalch equation
AB	=	actual measured bicarbonate (mEq/l)

Interpretation

$PaCO_2$ is expected to decrease 1.25 mmHg for each 1 mEq/l decrease in HCO_3. For practical purposes, the adult formula can be used in most circumstances at all ages.

Mixed disturbance

A lower than expected $PaCO_2$ suggests a superimposed respiratory alkalosis.* A higher than expected $PaCO_2$ suggests a superimposed respiratory acidosis.

* Infants with no significant respiratory distress or only mild CO_2 retention may overcompensate by crying during the blood letting, resulting in an insignificant superimposed acute respiratory alkalosis.

References

Ash MJ, Dell RB, Williams GSL, Cohen ML, Winters RW. Time course for the development of respiratory compensation in metabolic acidosis. *J Lab Clin Med* 1969; 73:610

Winters RW. Physiology of acid–base disorders. In Winters RW, ed. *The Body Fluids in Pediatrics*, 1st edn. Boston, MA: Little Brown, 1973:50–7

METABOLIC ALKALOSIS

Use

To identify the expected respiratory compensation in metabolic alkalosis, and to determine whether the imbalance exists alone (simple) or is accompanied by one or more additional acid–base disturbances (mixed). In acute states of metabolic alkalosis, respiratory compensation (although irregular and unpredictable) generally occurs quickly, and the $PaCO_2$ will reach expected levels in 4–6 h. For practical purposes, therefore, $PaCO_2$ should be considered a reflection of a steady state (acute *or* chronic state) of a simple or mixed disturbance.

Definition

> pH > 7.43
> HCO_3 more than 3.0 mEq/l above normal for age

Formulas for respiratory compensation

Adult: Expected $PaCO_2 = [0.6 \times (AB - 25)] + 40$

Child: Expected $PaCO_2 = [0.6 \times (AB - NB)] + NPaCO_2$

AB	=	actual measured bicarbonate (mEq/l)
NB	=	normal bicarbonate in infants and children (mEq/l) – refer to Henderson–Hasselbalch equation
$NPaCO_2$	=	normal $PaCO_2$ in infants and children (mmHg) – refer to Henderson–Hasselbalch equation

Interpretation

$PaCO_2$ will increase by 0.6–0.75 mmHg for each 1 mEq/l increase in HCO_3. This relationship exists in infants, children and adults. Also, the adult formula can be used in most circumstances throughout life.

Mixed disturbance

> A lower than expected increase in $PaCO_2$ suggests a superimposed respiratory alkalosis*
> A greater than expected increase in $PaCO_2$ suggests a superimposed respiratory acidosis

Metabolic alkalosis is always hypochloremic (normal anion gap). The imbalance can be either saline-responsive or saline-resistant. The responsive form is characterized by hypovolemia and a urine chloride level of < 20 mEq/l. The resistant form is associated with an increased extracellular volume, a urine chloride level of > 20 mEq/l, and is caused by excess mineralocorticoids with potassium wasting.

---

* Infants with no significant respiratory distress or only mild CO_2 retention may overcompensate by crying during the blood letting, resulting in an insignificant superimposed acute respiratory alkalosis.

References

Cogan MG. *Fluid and Electrolyte Physiology and Pathophysiology.* Norwalk, CT: Appleton & Lange, 1991:225:237–8

Winters RW. Physiology of acid–base disorders. In Winters RW, ed. *The Body Fluids in Pediatrics*, 1st edn. Boston, MA: Little Brown, 1973:57–61

RESPIRATORY ACIDOSIS

Use

To identify the expected metabolic compensation in respiratory acidosis, and to determine whether the imbalance exists alone (simple) or is accompanied by one or more additional acid–base disturbances (mixed). In sustained states of respiratory acidosis, maximal metabolic compensation by the kidneys occurs slowly, and the HCO_3 may not reach expected levels for 2–4 days. Interpretation of blood gases, therefore, is different for acute CO_2 retention than for chronic CO_2 retention.

Definition

> $pH < 7.35$
> $PaCO_2 > 3$ mmHg above normal for age

Formulas for expected metabolic compensation

Adult: Acute: Expected $HCO_3 = 25 + 0.1(PaCO_2 - 40)$
       Chronic: Expected $HCO_3 = 25 + 0.4(PaCO_2 - 40)$

Child: Acute: Expected $HCO_3 = NB + 0.1(PaCO_2 - NPaCO_2)$
       Chronic: Expected $HCO_3 = NB + 0.4(PaCO_2 - NPaCO_2)$

$PaCO_2$ =   arterial CO_2 tension (mmHg)
NB =   normal bicarbonate for age (mEq/l) – refer to Henderson–Hasselbalch equation
$NPaCO_2$ =   normal $PaCO_2$ for age (mmHg) – refer to Henderson–Hasselbalch equation

Formulas for expected pH change

$$\text{Acute: Expected decrease in pH} = \frac{0.08 \times (\text{measured } PaCO_2 - NPaCO_2)}{10}$$

$$\text{Chronic: Expected decrease in pH} = \frac{0.03 \times (\text{measured } PaCO_2 - NPaCO_2)}{10}$$

Interpretation

In acute respiratory acidosis (less than 24–48 h duration) HCO_3 will increase 0.1 mEq/l and pH will decrease 0.08 units for each 1.0 mmHg increase in $PaCO_2$. In chronic respiratory acidosis (over 48 h duration) HCO_3 will increase 0.4 mEq/l and pH will decrease 0.03 units for each 1.0 mmHg increase in $PaCO_2$.

Mixed disturbance

An increase in HCO_3 less than expected and a decrease in pH more than expected suggests a superimposed metabolic acidosis.
An increase in HCO_3 greater than expected and an increase in pH less than expected suggests a superimposed metabolic alkalosis.

Reference

Winters RW. Physiology of acid–base disorders. In Winters RW, ed. *The Body Fluids in Pediatrics*, 1st edn. Boston, MA: Little Brown, 1973:61–7

RESPIRATORY ALKALOSIS

Use

To identify the expected metabolic compensation in respiratory alkalosis, and to determine whether the imbalance exists alone (simple) or is accompanied by one or more additional acid–base disturbances (mixed). In sustained states of respiratory alkalosis, maximal metabolic compensation by the kidneys occurs slowly, and the HCO_3 may not reach expected levels for 2–4 days. Interpretation of blood gases, therefore, is different for acute hypocapnea than for chronic hypocapnea.

Definition

> pH > 7.43
> $PaCO_2$ > 3 mmHg below normal for age

Formulas for metabolic compensation

Adult: Acute: Expected $HCO_3 = 25 - 0.2(40 - PaCO_2)$
Chronic: Expected $HCO_3 = 25 - 0.4(40 - PaCO_2)$

Child: Acute: Expected $HCO_3 = NB - 0.2(NPaCO_2 - PaCO_2)$
Chronic: Expected $HCO_3 = NB - 0.4(NPaCO_2 - PaCO_2)$

$PaCO_2$ =   arterial CO_2 tension (mmHg)

NB   =   normal bicarbonate for age (mEq/l) – refer to Henderson–Hasselbalch equation

$NPaCO_2$ =   normal $PaCO_2$ for age (mmHg) – refer to Henderson–Hasselbalch equation

Formulas for expected pH change

$$\text{Acute: Expected increase in pH} = \frac{0.08 \times (NPaCO_2 - \text{measured } PaCO_2)}{10}$$

$$\text{Chronic: Expected increase in pH} = \frac{0.03 \times (NPaCO_2 - \text{measured } PaCO_2)}{10}$$

Interpretation

In acute respiratory alkalosis (less than 24–48 h duration) HCO_3 will decrease 0.2 mEq/l and pH will increase 0.08 units for each 1.0 mmHg decrease in $PaCO_2$. In chronic respiratory alkalosis (over 48 h duration) HCO_3 will decrease 0.4 mEq/l and pH will increase 0.03 units for each 1.0 mmHg decrease in $PaCO_2$.

Mixed disturbance

A decrease in HCO_3 less than expected and an increase in pH more than expected suggests a superimposed metabolic alkalosis.
A decrease in HCO_3 greater than expected and an increase in pH less than expected suggests a superimposed metabolic acidosis.

Note: HCO_3 does not fall below 16 mEq/l in respiratory alkalosis unless there is a coexisting metabolic acidosis (mixed disturbance).

References

Effros RM, Widell JL. Acid–base balance. In Murray JF, Nadel JA, eds. *Textbook of Respiratory Medicine*, 2nd edn. Philadelphia, PA: WB Saunders, 1994:175–98

Schwartz GJ. General principles of acid–base physiology. In Holliday MA, Barratt TM, Avner ED, eds. *Pediatric Nephrology*, 3rd edn. Baltimore, MD: Williams & Wilkins, 1994:225

Winters RW. Physiology of acid–base disorders. In Winters RW, ed. *The Body Fluids in Pediatrics*. 1st edn. Boston, MA: Little Brown, 1973:67–71

ANION GAP – SERUM

Use

To distinguish between normal and elevated serum anion gap. Although normal anion gap acidosis is usually accompanied by hyperchloremia, an accompanying hyponatremia may shift the chloride concentration into the normal range while maintaining a normal anion gap.

Formula

$$AG = Na - (HCO_3 + Cl)$$

AG	=	anion gap (mEq/l)
Na	=	serum sodium (mEq/l)
HCO_3	=	serum bicarbonate (mEq/l)
Cl	=	serum chloride (mEq/l)

Interpretation

Normal anion gap = 12 ± 2 mEq/l

An elevated anion gap indicates an increase in the circulating unmeasured anions (see table below).
A low anion gap indicates a decrease in unmeasured anions (usually low protein), or an increase in cations (i.e. hypercalcemia, hypermagnesemia or hypergammaglobulinemia).

Comparison between normal anion gap and elevated anion gap in metabolic acidosis

Normal anion gap (loss of HCO_3)	Elevated anion gap (gain of strong acid)
Gastrointestinal (diarrhea)	Ketoacids (diabetes, starvation)
Renal (tubular acidosis)	Lactic acid (hypoxemia, metabolic error)
	Organic acids (metabolic error)
	Mineral acids (uremia)
	Exogenous acids (toxins)

References

Brensilver JM, Goldberger E. *A Primer of Water, Electrolyte, and Acid–Base Syndromes*, 8th edn. Philadelphia, PA: FA Davis, 1996:13

Schwartz GJ. General principles of acid–base physiology. In Holliday MA, Barratt TM, Avner ED, eds. *Pediatric Nephrology*, 3rd edn. Baltimore, MD: Williams & Wilkins, 1994:224

Winters RW. Physiology of acid–base disorders. In Winters RW, ed. *The Body Fluids in Pediatrics*, 1st edn. Boston, MA: Little Brown, 1973:51

ANION GAP – URINE

Use

To evaluate the role of kidney tubular function in the pathogenesis of a normal serum anion gap acidosis.

Formula

$$UAG = Na_u + K_u - Cl_u$$

UAG	=	Urinary anion gap (mEq/l)
Na_u	=	Urinary sodium concentration (mEq/l)
K_u	=	Urinary potassium concentration (mEq/l)
Cl_u	=	Urinary chloride concentration (mEq/l)

Interpretation

Mean urinary anion gap is less than -31 mEq/l in children with significant acidosis. Values of UAG which are positive (above zero) are generally considered abnormal. A normal UAG should be present with hyperchloremic (normal anion gap) metabolic acidosis due to gastrointestinal bicarbonate loss in the presence of normal kidney tubules that are producing NH_3, which diffuses into the filtrate, binds H^+ and is excreted as NH_4^+. A positive UAG reflects low renal NH_3 production and suggests that the acidosis may be caused by a renal tubular disorder (e.g. renal tubular acidosis).

References

Carlisle EJ, Donnelly SM, Halperin ML. Renal tubular acidosis (RTA): recognize the ammonium defect and pH or get the urine pH. *Pediatr Nephrol* 1991;5:242–8

Goldstein MB, Bear R, Richarson RM, Marston PA, Halperin ML. The urine anion gap, a clinically useful index of ammonia excretion. *Am J Med Sci* 1986;292:198–202

Rodriguiz-Soriano J. Tubular disorders of electrolyte regulation. In Holliday MA, Barratt TM, Avner ED, eds. *Pediatric Nephrology*, 3rd edn. Baltimore, MD: Williams & Wilkins, 1994:224

BLOOD GASES

ARTERIAL OXYGEN CONTENT OF WHOLE BLOOD

Use

To calculate the O_2 content of whole blood as a function of the hemoglobin concentration, O_2 saturation of hemoglobin and the arterial O_2 tension. This formula reflects the relative contributions of hemoglobin and plasma in the O_2-carrying capacity of whole blood.

Formula

$$O_2C = \left(1.34 \times Hb \times \frac{SaO_2}{100}\right) + (0.0031 \times PaO_2)$$

O_2C	=	oxygen content of blood (ml/dl or vol%)
Hb	=	hemoglobin concentration (g/dl)
SaO_2	=	saturation of hemoglobin in blood (%)
PaO_2	=	partial pressure of oxygen in plasma (mmHg)
1.34	=	ml O_2 per gram of fully saturated hemoglobin (ml/g)
0.0031	=	ml O_2 dissolved in 100 ml plasma per mmHg of PaO_2 (ml/mmHg/dl)

Note: The neonate is born with an average of 70% fetal hemoglobin. While oxygen content of saturated fetal hemoglobin is the same as for adult hemoglobin, saturation of total hemoglobin in infants is higher for any given PaO_2. (See oxyhemoglobin dissociation curve.)

References

Delivoria-Papadopoulos M, Roncevic NP, Oski FA. Postnatal changes in oxygen transport of term, premature, and sick infants: the role of red cell 2,3-DPG and adult hemoglobin. *Pediatr Res* 1971;5:235

Gutierrez G, Price K. Abnormalities of oxygen delivery and uptake in sepsis. In Carlson RW, Gehab MA, eds. *Principles and Practice of Medical Intensive Care.* Philadelphia, PA: WB Saunders, 1993:359

Weinberger SE, Drazen JM. Disturbances of respiratory function. In Fauci AS, Braunwald E, Isselbacher KJ, Wilson JD, Martin JB, Kasper DL, Hauser SL, Longo DL, eds. *Harrison's Principles of Internal Medicine*, 14th edn. New York, NY: McGraw-Hill, 1998:1414

OXYHEMOGLOBIN DISSOCIATION CURVE

Use

To determine the percent saturation of hemoglobin with oxygen at varying oxygen tensions.

Formula

$$\%O_2\ Sat = \cfrac{1}{\left[\cfrac{23\ 400}{(PO_2)^3 + (150 \times PO_2)} + 1\right]} \times 100 = \frac{100\left[(PO_2)^3 + (150\ PO_2)\right]}{23\ 400 + (PO_2)^3 + (150\ PO_2)}$$

$$PO_2 \quad = \quad \text{arterial oxygen tension (mmHg)}$$

Definitions in blood gas measurement

(1) Oxygen content (volume %, ml/100 ml) = volume of oxygen that 100 ml of blood contains
(2) Oxygen tension = partial pressure of oxygen in blood (mmHg)
(3) Oxygen capacity = volume of oxygen taken up by hemoglobin when exposed to high O_2 tensions
(4) Oxygen saturation (%) = percent of hemoglobin saturated with oxygen

$$= \frac{content\ (\%)}{capacity\ (\%)} \times 100$$

Note: The neonate is born with an average of 70% fetal hemoglobin. While oxygen content of saturated fetal hemoglobin is the same as for adult hemoglobin, saturation of total hemoglobin in infants is higher for any given PO_2. This is so because the presence of fetal hemoglobin increases the red blood cells' affinity for O_2, which shifts the oxyhemoglobin dissociation curve to the left. Fetal hemoglobin falls to less than 2% at 6 months of age, after which time oxygen content varies with hemoglobin levels and otherwise mimics adult values.

References

Cotes JE. *Lung Function, Assessment, and Application in Medicine*, 5th edn. London: Blackwell, 1993:280–1

Delivoria-Papadopoulos M, Roncevic NP, Oski FA. Postnatal changes in oxygen transport of term, premature, and sick infants: the role of red cell 2,3-DPG and adult hemoglobin. *Pediatr Res* 1971;5:235

O'Brodovich HM, Haddad GG. The functional basis of respiratory pathology. In Chernick VC, Kendig EL Jr, eds. *Kendig's Disorders of the Respiratory Tract in Children*, 5th edn. Philadelphia, PA: WB Saunders, 1990:30–3

Ohls RK, Christensen RD. Development of the hematopoietic system. In Behrman RE, Kliegman RM, Jenson HB, eds. *Nelson Textbook of Pediatrics*, 16th edn. Philadelphia, PA: WB Saunders, 2000:1458–60

Pearson HA. Origin and development of blood cells and coagulation factors. In Miller DR, Pearson HA, Baehner RL, McMillan CW, eds. *Smith's Blood Diseases of Infancy and Childhood*, 4th edn. St Louis, MO: CV Mosby, 1978:16–17

Severinghaus JW. Simple, accurate equations for human blood O_2 dissociation computations. *J Appl Physiol*, 1979;46:599–602

HEMOGLOBIN OXYGEN SATURATION

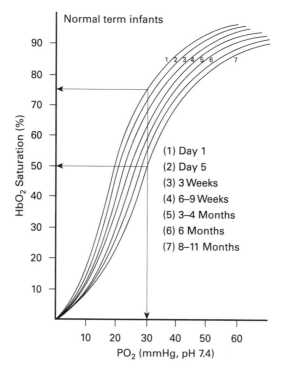

Infant oxyhemoglobin dissociation curve

Term infant hemoglobin oxygen dissociation curve varies with age. The arrows indicate that, at an O_2 pressure of 30 mmHg, hemoglobin is 75% saturated in the 1-day-old, and 50% saturated in the 8-month-old. The 50% saturation (P_{50}) O_2 pressure in a normal adult is 27 mmHg. (From Deliveria-Papadopoulos M, *et al. Pediatr Res* 1971;5:235)

BODY METRICS

BODY WATER COMPARTMENTS

Use

To calculate volumes of water compartments as a function of age, weight and gender.

Formulas

Children over 1 year:

$$\text{TBW} = 0.61 \times \text{Wt} + 0.251$$
$$\text{ECF} = 0.239 \times \text{Wt} + 0.325$$

TBW	=	total body water (liters)
ECF	=	extracellular fluid (liters)
Wt	=	weight (kg)

	Percent body weight		
Distribution of body water	*Birth*	*1 year*	*Adult*
Plasma water	4.5	4.5	4.5
Interstitial fluid	40.5	20.5	15.5
Extracellular fluid	45	25	20
Intracellular fluid	30	40	40
Total body water	75	65	60
Blood volume	9.5	7.5	7.8

Note: Women and obese children have less total body water, as low as 50–55% of body weight.

References

Adelman RD, Solhaug MJ. Pathophysiology of body fluids and fluid therapy. In Behrman RE, Kliegman RM, Jenson HB, eds. *Nelson Textbook of Pediatrics*, 16th edn. Philadelphia, PA: WB Saunders, 2000:189–90

Winters RW. Regulation of normal water and electrolyte metabolism. In Winters RW, ed. *The Body Fluids in Pediatrics*, 1st edn. Boston, MA: Little Brown, 1973:99–101

BODY SURFACE AREA

Use

To estimate body surface area from weight and height.

Formulas

$BSA = 0.007184 \times Wt^{0.425} \times Ht^{0.725}$ (Dubois formula)
or

$$BSA = \sqrt{\frac{Ht \times Wt}{3600}} \text{ (Mosteller's formula)}$$

or
$BSA = Wt^{0.5378} \times Ht^{0.3964} \times 0.024265$ (Haycock, Schwartz, Wisotsky formula)

BSA	=	body surface area (m²)
Wt	=	weight (kg)
Ht	=	height (cm)

Note: For infants and children the Haycock or Mosteller formula is preferable.

References

Dubois D, Dubois EF. A formula to estimate the approximate surface area if height and weight be known. *Arch Intern Med* 1916;17:863–71

Haycock GB, Schwartz GJ, Wisotsky DH. Geometric method for measuring body surface area: a height–weight formula validated in infants, children, and adults. *J Pediatr* 1978;93:62–6

Preece MA. Evaluation of growth and development. In Holliday MA, Barratt TM, Avner ED, eds. *Pediatric Nephrology*, 3rd edn. Baltimore, MD: Williams & Wilkins, 1994:391

BODY MASS INDEX

Use

To evaluate the status of body fat storage and relative obesity.

Formula

$$BMI = \frac{Wt}{Ht^2}$$

BMI	=	body mass index (kg/m²)
Wt	=	weight (kg)
Ht	=	height (cm)

Interpretation

Optimal BMI	=	< 75th centile
Overweight	=	≥ 90th centile
Obese	=	≥ 95th centile

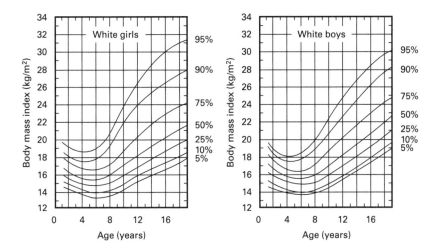

Example for boys and girls aged 10 years

	BMI (kg/m²)	
Status	*Boys*	*Girls*
Optimal	< 18.5	< 19.0
Overweight	≥ 20.3	≥ 22.0
Obese	≥ 22.2	≥ 24.0

Note: Mean BMI values are slightly higher for Black and Hispanic girls than for white girls.

References

Hammer LD, Kramer HC, Wilson DM, *et al.* Standardized percentile curves of body mass index for children and adolescents. *Am J Dis Child* 1991;145:259

Rosner B, Prineas R, Loggie J, Daniels SR. Percentiles for body mass index in U.S. children 5 to 17 years of age. *J Pediatr* 1998;132:211–22

UPPER/LOWER RATIO

Use

To identify short-limb dwarfism and other bone disorders.

Formula

$$\text{U/L ratio} = \frac{\text{UBS}}{\text{LBS}}$$

U/L ratio = ratio of upper body segment to lower body segment
LBS = lower body segment, defined as distance from symphysis pubis to floor
UBS = upper body segment, defined as height minus lower body segment

Interpretation

	Normal values		
	Birth	3 years	Over 7 years
U/L ratio	1.7	1.3	1.0

Reference

Needlman RD. Growth and development. In Behrman RE, Kliegman RM, Jenson HB, eds. *Nelson Textbook of Pediatrics*, 16th edn. Philadelphia, PA: WB Saunders, 2000:59

IDEAL BODY WEIGHT AND HEIGHT IN CHILDREN

Use

To estimate ideal body weight and height for age in infants and children

Wt_i = ideal body weight (kg)
Ht_i = ideal height (cm)
A_{yr} = age in years
A_{mo} = age in months

Ideal weight: infants aged 0–24 months

	0–6 months	6–12 months	12–24 months
Infant boys	$Wt_i = 0.733 A_{mo} + 3.6$	$Wt_i = 0.433 A_{mo} + 5.4$	$Wt_i = 0.183 A_{mo} + 8.4$
Infant girls	$Wt_i = 0.667 A_{mo} + 3.4$	$Wt_i = 0.400 A_{mo} + 5.0$	$Wt_i = 0.183 A_{mo} + 7.6$

Ideal weight: children and young adults aged 2–20 years

	2–10 years	10–16 years	16–20 years
Boys	$Wt_i = 2.25 A_{yr} + 8.50$	$Wt_i = 5.00 A_{yr} + 19.0$	$Wt_i = 2.25 A_{yr} + 25$
Girls	$Wt_i = 2.38 A_{yr} + 7.25$	$Wt_i = 3.17 A_{yr} + 3.33$	$Wt_i = A_{yr} + 38$

Ideal length: infants aged 0–24 months

	0–6 months	6–12 months	12–24 months
Infant boys	$Ht_i = 2.67 A_{mo} + 52$	$Ht_i = 1.33 A_{mo} + 60$	$Ht_i = A_{mo} + 64$
Infant girls	$Ht_i = 2.33 A_{mo} + 52$	$Ht_i = 1.50 A_{mo} + 57$	$Ht_i = 0.92 A_{mo} + 64$

Ideal height: children and young adults aged 2–20 years

	2–14 years	14–20 years
Boys	$Ht_i = 6.417 A_{yr} + 76$	$Ht_i = 2.167 A_{yr} + 137$
Girls	$Ht_i = 5.143 A_{yr} + 86$	$Ht_i = 0.500 A_{yr} + 153$

Interpretation

These linear equations were derived from growth charts revised in November 2000. The computed values of ideal weight and height generally approximate the 50th centile, and in no instance fall above or below the 75th or 25th centile, respectively.

Reference

National Center for Health Statistics in collaboration with the National Center for Chronic Disease Prevention and Health Promotion, revised and corrected November 21, 2000

CARDIOVASCULAR SYSTEM

BLOOD PRESSURE

Use

To define the upper limits of normal blood pressure for children and adolescents from 1 to 18 years.

Formulas

$SBP = 1.8A + 110$

$DBP = A + 73$

SBP	=	systolic blood pressure (mmHg)
DBP	=	diastolic blood pressure (mmHg)
A	=	age (years)

Interpretation

The formulas define the upper limits of normal blood pressure (95th centile) for children and adolescents from ages 1 to 18 years. While girls have some-what lower pressures than boys, estimates derived by these formulas are close to the upper limits of normal for both sexes. Patients with values exceeding these pressures are considered to have significant hypertension.

The following table defines the 95th centile blood pressures in infants under 1 year of age for boys, with values for girls in parentheses

Blood pressure of infants

	Birth	3 months	6 months	9 months	12 months
Systolic	92 (85)	110 (108)	110 (110)	110 (110)	110 (110)
Diastolic	72 (72)	67 (68)	70 (69)	73 (70)	74 (72)

Mean arterial pressure in prematures can be estimated by: gestational age (in weeks) + 5.
Significant hypertension in prematures can be considered to be defined by a mean arterial pressure of ≥ gestational age (in weeks) + 15.

References

Report of the Second Task Force on Blood Pressure Control in Children. *Pediatrics* 1987;79:7

Yetman RJ, Bonilla-Felix MA, Portman RJ. Primary hypertension in children and adolescents. In: Holliday MA, Barratt TM, Avner ED, eds. *Pediatric Nephrology*, 3rd edn. Baltimore, MD: Williams & Wilkins, 1994:1117–45

Zubrow AB, Hulman S, Kushner H, *et al*. Determinants of blood pressure in infants admitted to neonatal intensive care units: a prospective multicenter study. *J Perinatol* 1995;15:470–9

CARDIAC INDEX AND STROKE INDEX

Use

To evaluate cardiac output. These formulas require direct measurements of cardiac output and stroke volumes. Correction of measured values for body surface area yields the corresponding indices.

Cardiac index

Formula

$$CI = \frac{CO}{BSA}$$

CI = cardiac index (liters/min/m^2)
CO = cardiac output (liters/min)
BSA = body surface area (m^2)

Stroke index

Formula

$$SI = \frac{CO}{BSA \times R} \times 1000$$

SI = stroke index (ml/m^2)
CO = cardiac output (liters/min)
BSA = body surface area (m^2)
R = heart rate (beats/min)

Interpretation

Normal values

Age	Cardiac index (l/min/m^2)	Resting heart rate (beats/min)	Stroke index (ml/m^2)
Birth	5.0–5.5	123	40–45
2 months	2.5–5.0	110	23–45
Adult	2.5–5.0	60	42–50

At birth CO is about twice as high as adult values when factored by surface area (i.e. CI), and 4–5 times higher when factored by weight. By 2 months of age values of CI in liters/min/m^2 are near adult values.

Stroke index likewise varies with age. Since heart rates are high in the neonate, the SI is near adult norms. The SI may fall in the first 2 months to near half adult norms because of a relative tachycardia in infants.

References

Bernstein D. Developmental biology of the cardiovascular system. In Behrman RE, Kliegman RM, Jenson HB, eds. *Nelson Textbook of Pediatrics*, 16th edn. Philadelphia, PA: WB Saunders, 2000:1341–2

Freed MD. Invasive diagnostic and therapeutic techniques. In Adams FH, Emmanouilides GC, Riemenschneider TA, eds. *Moss' Heart Disease in Infants, Children, and Adolescents*, 4th edn. Baltimore, MD: Williams & Wilkins, 1989:136–8

CARDIAC OUTPUT – FICK PRINCIPLE

Use

To estimate cardiac output using oxygen uptake as an indicator.

Formulas

$$CO = \frac{ConsO_2}{ContAO_2 - ContVO_2} \times 100$$

CO	=	cardiac output (liters/min)
$ConsO_2$	=	oxygen consumption (ml/min)
$ContAO_2$	=	arterial oxygen content (ml/liter)
$ContVO_2$	=	venous oxygen content (ml/liter)

$$CI = \frac{CO}{BSA}$$

CI	=	cardiac index (liter/min/m^2)
BSA	=	body surface area (m^2)

Interpretation

Normal values

Age	Cardiac Index (*l/min/m²*)
Birth	5.0–5.5
2 months	2.5–5.0
Adult	2.5–5.0

See 'Cardiac index' and 'Stroke index' for comment.

The Fick Principle states that the uptake of a substance by an organ is the product of blood flow and the arteriovenous (A-V) differences across the organ. In the case of Fick cardiac output, the substance is oxygen and the organ is the lung. The venous blood is sampled from the pulmonary artery, and the arterial blood is sampled peripherally. The blood O_2 content (vol%) is calculated from saturation (%) × hemoglobin (g/dl) × 1.36. The O_2 consumption is measure by collecting expired air. More convenient dye and thermodilution methods have largely replaced the Fick method.

References

Bernstein D. Developmental biology of the cardiovascular system. In Behrman RE, Kliegman RM, Jenson HB, eds. *Nelson Textbook of Pediatrics*, 16th edn. Philadelphia, PA: WB Saunders, 2000:1359–60

Freed MD. Invasive diagnostic and therapeutic techniques. In Adams FH, Emmanouilides GC, Riemenschneider TA, eds. *Moss' Heart Disease in Infants, Children, and Adolescents*, 4th edn. Baltimore, MD: Williams & Wilkins, 1989:136–8

Grossman W. Cardiac catheterization. In Braunwald E, ed. *Heart Disease: A Textbook of Cardiovascular Medicine*, 4th edn. Philadelphia, PA: WB Saunders, 1992:180–203

CORRECTED QT INTERVAL

Use

Corrects the electrocardiographic QT interval for heart rate and for age. The QT interval is a measure of ventricular depolarization (QRS) plus repolarization (ST).

Formula

$$QT_c = \frac{QT}{\sqrt{RR}}$$

QT_c	=	corrected QT interval (s)
QT	=	measured QT interval (s)
RR	=	measured RR interval (s)

Derivation of RR and √RR from heart rate

Heart rate (bpm)	RR (s)	$\sqrt{RR}$
60	1.000	1.000
65	0.923	0.961
70	0.857	0.926
75	0.800	0.894
80	0.750	0.866
85	0.706	0.840
90	0.667	0.816
95	0.632	0.795
100	0.600	0.775
105	0.571	0.756
110	0.545	0.739
115	0.522	0.722
120	0.500	0.707

Interpretation

Normal QT_c

Age	QT_c (s)
3–4 days	≤ 0.44
< 6 months	≤ 0.45
Children	≤ 0.44
Adolescents	≤ 0.425
Adult males	≤ 0.39–0.44
Adult females	≤ 0.43–0.46

Prolonged QT_c can be congenital or can be acquired as a result of ischemic heart disease, cardiomyopathy, electrolyte abnormalities, drugs, etc. A shortened QT_c occurs with hyperkalemia, digitalis, hypercalcemia and acidosis.

References

Fisch C. Electrocardiography and vectorcardiography. In Braunwald E, ed. *Heart Disease: A Textbook of Cardiovascular Medicine*, 4th edn. Philadelphia, PA: WB Saunders, 1992:116–60

Park MK. *Pediatric Cardiology for Practitioners*, 3rd edn. St Louis, MO: Mosby, 1996:34–43

Schwartz PJ, Stramba-Badiale M, Segantini A, *et al*. Prolongation of the QT interval and the sudden infant death syndrome. *N Engl J Med* 1998;338:1709–14

Walsh EP. Electrocardiography and introduction to electrophysiologic techniques. In Flyer DC, ed. *Nadas' Pediatric Cardiology*. Philadelphia, PA: Hanley & Belfus, 1992:128

MEAN ARTERIAL PRESSURE

Use

To estimate mean arterial pressure without the need for direct intra-arterial monitoring.

Formula

$$MAP = DP + \frac{SP - DP}{3}$$

MAP	=	mean arterial pressure (mmHg)
DP	=	diastolic pressure (mmHg)
SP	=	systolic pressure (mmHg)

Interpretation

Significant hypertension using mean arterial pressure

Age	MAP
Birth	≥ 74
30 days	≥ 77
1–24 months	≥ 87
3–5 years	≥ 89
6–9 years	≥ 93
10–12 years	≥ 97
13–15 years	≥ 103
16–18 years	≥ 109

Significant hypertension over 1 month of age based on MAP can be defined using the following formula:

$$MAP > 1.222A + 87$$

A = age (years)

Average MAP in prematures can be estimated by: gestational age (in weeks) + 5.
Significant hypertension in prematures can be considered as defined by a MAP ≥ gestational age (in weeks) + 15.

References

Report of the Second Task Force on Blood Pressure Control in Children – 1987. *Pediatrics* 1987;79:1–25

Yetman RJ, Bonilla-Felix MA, Portman RJ. Primary hypertension in children and adolescents. In Holliday MA, Barratt TM, Avner ED, eds. *Pediatric Nephrology*, 3rd edn. Baltimore, MD: Williams & Wilkins, 1994:1117–45

Zubrow AB, Hulman S, Kushner H, *et al*. Determinants of blood pressure in infants admitted to neonatal intensive care units: a prospective multicenter study. *J Perinatol* 1995;15:470–9

SYSTEMIC VASCULAR RESISTANCE AND INDEX

Use

To estimate systemic vascular resistance.

Formula

$$SVR = \frac{MAP - CVP}{CO} \times 80$$

SVR	=	systemic vascular resistance (dyne/s/cm^{-5})
MAP	=	mean arterial pressure (mmHg)
CVP	=	central venous pressure (mmHg)
CO	=	cardiac output (liters/min)

Interpretation

Normal SVR = 1170 ± 270 dyne/s/cm^{-5} (remains constant throughout childhood)

Systemic vascular resistance index

$$SVRI = SVR \times BSA$$

SVRI	=	systemic vascular resistance index (dyne/s/cm^{-5}/m^2)
SVR	=	systemic vascular resistance (dyne/s/cm^{-5})
BSA	=	body surface area (m^2)

Interpretation

Normal SVRI obviously varies with surface area and, in pediatric patients, can be estimated by:

SVRI (dyne/s/cm^{-5}/m^2) = 6658/CI + 158, where CI is cardiac index (l/min/m^2).

References

Freed MD. Invasive diagnostic and therapeutic techniques. In Adams FH, Emmanouilides GC, Riemenschneider TA, eds. *Moss' Heart Disease in Infants, Children, and Adolescents*, 4th edn. Baltimore, MD: Williams & Wilkins, 1989:144,325

Grossman W. Cardiac catheterization. In Braunwald E, ed. *Heart Disease: A Textbook of Cardiovascular Medicine*, 4th edn. Philadelphia, PA: WB Saunders, 1992: 180–203

Lock JE, Einzig S, Moller JH. Hemodynamic responses to exercise in normal children. *Am J Cardiol* 1978;41:1278–84

PULMONARY VASCULAR RESISTANCE

Use

To estimate pulmonary vascular resistance.

Formula

$$PVR = \frac{PA - PCW}{CO} \times 80$$

PVR	=	pulmonary vascular resistance (dyne/s/cm^{-5})
PA	=	mean pulmonary artery pressure (mmHg)
PCW	=	pulmonary capillary wedge pressure or left atrial pressure (mmHg)
CO	=	cardiac output (l/min)

Interpretation

Normal PVR varies with age. The value is near systemic vascular resistance at birth. It falls rapidly in the first few days of life, less rapidly after the first 1–2 months, and continues to fall slowly until reaching near adult values by 10 years. Representative values are listed in the table.

Age	PVR (dyne/s/cm^{-5})
Birth	1500
2 years	600
3 years	400
10 years	150
Adult	20–130

References

Freed MD. Invasive diagnostic and therapeutic techniques. In Adams FH, Emmanouilides GC, Riemenschneider TA, eds. *Moss' Heart Disease in Infants, Children, and Adolescents*, 4th edn. Baltimore, MD: Williams & Wilkins 1989: 144, 325

Grossman W. Cardiac catheterization. In Braunwald E, ed. *Heart Disease: A Textbook of Cardiovascular Medicine*, 4th edn. Philadelphia, PA: WB Saunders, 1992: 180–203

Kulik TJ. Pulmonary hypertension. In Fyler DC, ed. *Nadas' Pediatric Cardiology*. Philadelphia, PA: Hanley & Belfus, 1992:84–5

Lock JE, Einzig S, Moller JH. Hemodynamic responses to exercise in normal children. *Am J Cardiol* 1978;41:1278–84

PULMONARY/SYSTEMIC FLOW RATIO

Use

To estimate the relative magnitude of right-to-left or left-to-right shunting in congenital heart disease.

Formula

$$P:S\ ratio = \frac{O_2Cao - O_2Cmv}{O_2Cpv - O_2Cpa} : 1$$

P : S ratio	=	pulmonary to systemic blood flow ratio
O_2Cao	=	O_2 content (ml/l) in aorta
O_2Cmv	=	O_2 content (ml/l) in mixed venous blood (SVC or right atrium)
O_2Cpv	=	O_2 content (ml/l) in pulmonary vein
O_2Cpa	=	O_2 content (ml/l) in pulmonary artery

Interpretation

A P : S ratio of 1 : 1 indicates no shunting. A value of 2 : 1 would indicate that blood flow from a left-to-right shunt was equal to systemic blood flow, and a likely surgical candidate. A value of 0.8 : 1 would indicate that pulmonary blood flow is 20% less than systemic flow because of a right-to-left shunt, a level seen in a cyanotic patient.

Reference

Park MK. *Pediatric Cardiology for Practitioners*, 3rd edn. St Louis, MO: Mosby, 1996:83–4

LEFT VENTRICLE SHORTENING FRACTION

Use

To measure left ventricular systolic function.

Formula

$$SF = \frac{LVED - LVES}{LVED} \times 100$$

SF = shortening fraction (%)
LVED = left ventricle end-diastolic dimension (cm)
LVES = left ventricle end-systolic dimension (cm)

Interpretation

This measurement represents the percent change of the difference from end-diastolic dimension to end-systolic dimension, normalized by the end-diastolic dimension. The measurement is generally made using the M-mode recording derived from a two-dimensional echocardiogram image. Values between 28% and 40% are considered normal.

Reference

Meyer RA. Echocardiography. In Adams FH, Emmanouilides GC, Riemenschneider TA, eds. *Moss' Heart Disease in Infants, Children, and Adolescents*, 4th edn. Baltimore, MD: Williams & Wilkins, 1989:259–60

ELECTROLYTES AND WATER

MAINTENANCE FLUIDS

Use

To estimate the maintenance fluid requirement for an average hospitalized infant or child.

Formulas

For body weight 0–10 kg

$$ML_{24} = Wt \times 100$$

For body weight 10–20 kg

$$ML_{24} = 1000 + [(Wt - 10) \times 50]$$

For body weight > 20 kg

$$ML_{24} = 1500 + [(Wt - 20) \times 20]$$

$$
\begin{aligned}
ML_{24} &= & \text{ml/24 h} \\
Wt &= & \text{body weight (kg)}
\end{aligned}
$$

Interpretation

The estimation of calories expended forms the basis of determining the maintenance caloric needs for hospitalized infants and children. It also forms the basis of determining the maintenance fluid requirements. The number of calories expended is equal to the number of milliliters of fluid required to replace the average urinary and insensible water losses (evaporative loss from skin and respiration) minus preformed water (water of oxidation and tissue catabolism).

The maintenance requirements for sodium and potassium are 2–4 mEq/100 ml each, which is added to the calculated fluid requirement. The composition of anions is dependent on the acid–base status of the patient.

References

Adelman RD, Solhaug MJ. Pathophysiology of body fluids and fluid therapy. In Behrman RE, Kleigman RM, Jenson HB, eds. *Nelson Textbook of Pediatrics*, 16th edn. Philadelphia, PA: WB Saunders, 2000:211–18

Holliday MA, Segar WE. *Parenteral Fluid Therapy*. Indianapolis, IN: Indiana University Medical Center, 1956:2–12

Holliday MA, Segar WE. The maintenance need for water in parenteral fluid therapy. *Pediatrics* 1957;19:823–32

Holliday MA. Fluid therapy. In Holliday MA, Barratt TM, Avner ED, eds. *Pediatric Nephrology*, 3rd edn. Baltimore, MD: Williams & Wilkins, 1994:295

DEFICIT FLUIDS

Use

To estimate the deficit fluid requirement in dehydration.

Formulas

$ML_{24} = PD \times Wt \times 10$

ML_{24}	=	ml/24 h
PD	=	percent dehydration
Wt	=	body weight (kg)

Interpretation

The estimation of degree of dehydration is generally based on clinical findings, and can usually be categorized as mild, moderate or severe. The relationship between the percent of body weight lost and the degree of dehydration varies somewhat with age (see table).

Percent dehydration (PD)

Age	Mild dehydration (%)	Moderate dehydration (%)	Severe dehydration (%)
Infants and small children	5	10	15
Older children and adults	3	6	9

The electrolyte composition of the deficit fluids (not including maintenance fluids) will depend on the associated conditions, as seen in the following:

31

Electrolyte losses per 100 ml of water lost by dehydration

Characteristics of condition	Composition of deficit fluid required		
	Na (mEq)	*K (mEq)**	*Cl (mEq)*
Isonatremia (Na 130–150 mEq/l)	8	6	6
Hyponatremia (Na <130 mEq/l)	10	8	10
Hypernatremia (Na >150 mEq/l)	2	2	– 4 to 0
Pyloric stenosis	8	10	10
Diabetic acidosis	8	6	6

* Generally potassium deficits cannot be replaced in 24 h IV fluids since potassium concentrations should not exceed 40 mEq/l under normal circumstances.

References

Adelman RD, Solhaug MJ. Pathophysiology of body fluids and fluid therapy. In Behrman RE, Kleigman RM, Jenson HB, eds. *Nelson Textbook of Pediatrics*, 16th edn. Philadelphia, PA: WB Saunders, 2000:211–18

Hellerstein S. Fluids and electrolytes: clinical aspects. *Pediatr Rev* 1993;14:103–15

Holliday MA, Segar WE. *Parenteral Fluid Therapy*. Indianapolis, IN: Indiana University Medical Center, 1956:2–12

Holliday MA, Segar WE. The maintenance need for water in parenteral fluid therapy. *Pediatrics* 1957;19:823–32

Holliday MA. Fluid therapy. In Holliday MA, Barratt TM, Avner ED, eds. *Pediatric Nephrology*, 3rd edn. Baltimore, MD: Williams & Wilkins, 1994:295

Oski FA. *Principles and Practice of Pediatrics*. Philadelphia, PA: JB Lippincott, 1994

HYPONATREMIA – FREE WATER EXCESS

Use

To calculate the excess total body water causing dilutional hyponatremia (sodium < 130 mEq/l).

Formula

$$FWE = \left(1 - \frac{Na}{140}\right) \times Wt \times F \times 1000$$

FWE = free water excess (ml)
Na = serum sodium concentration (mEq/l)
Wt = body weight (kg)
F = fraction of total body weight that is water

Age	Birth	1 year	Adult male	Adult female
Water fraction of total weight	0.75	0.65	0.60	0.50

Interpretation

This formula estimates free water excess only when there is no change in total body sodium, as in water intoxication and hypervolemia. Therapeutic correction by the administration of sodium is not advisable unless there are neurological manifestations. The treatment of choice with normal kidney function is water restriction in the face of a natural renal diuresis. Water restriction is also the treatment of choice in the syndrome of inappropriate antidiuretic hormone (SIADH) to allow for evaporative and renal water losses to correct the hyponatremia.

References

Adelman RD, Solhaug MJ. Pathophysiology of body fluids and fluid therapy. In Behrman RE, Kliegman RM, Jenson HB, eds. *Nelson Textbook of Pediatrics*, 16th edn. Philadelphia, PA: WB Saunders, 2000:189–90

Avner ED. Clinical disorders of water metabolism: hyponatremia and hypernatremia. *Pediatr Ann* 1995;24:23–7

Winters RW. Regulation of normal water and electrolyte metabolism. In Winters RW, ed. *The Body Fluids in Pediatrics*, 1st edn. Boston, MA: Little Brown, 1973:99–101

HYPONATREMIA – DEHYDRATION

Use

To calculate the pure sodium deficit causing hyponatremia (sodium < 130 mEq/l) in a dehydrated patient.

$$PSD = (140 - Na) \times Wt \times F$$

PSD	=	pure sodium deficit (mEq)
Na	=	serum sodium concentration (mEq/l)
Wt	=	body weight (kg)
F	=	fraction of body weight that is water

Age	Birth	1 year	Adult male	Adult female
Water fraction of total weight	0.75	0.65	0.60	0.50

Interpretation

This formula estimates the sodium deficit in excess of the isotonic losses from dehydration. The implication is that the sodium losses are disproportionately greater than the water losses. Therapeutic correction of the serum sodium concentration is best performed slowly over 48 h. A correction of < 10 mEq/l per day is recommended. Rapid correction has resulted in central pontine myelinolysis, a serious central nervous complication, but this condition is rare in children.

When serum sodium concentrations are below 120 mEq/l, or when seizures are present, the following formula may be used to estimate the number of milliequivalents of sodium to provide a more rapid correction to raise the serum sodium concentration to 120 mEq/l. This can be accomplished with 3% NaCl (approximately 0.5 mEq/ml) over 4 h.

$$mEqNa = (120 - Na) \times Wt \times F$$

References

Adelman RD, Solhaug MJ. Pathophysiology of body fluids and fluid therapy. In Behrman RE, Kliegman RM, Jenson HB, eds. *Nelson Textbook of Pediatrics*, 16th edn. Philadelphia, PA: WB Saunders, 2000:189–90

Avner ED. Clinical disorders of water metabolism: hyponatremia and hypernatremia. *Pediatr Ann* 1995;24:23–7

Holliday MA. Fluid and nutrition support. In Holliday MA, Barratt TM, Avner ED, eds. *Pediatric Nephrology*, 3rd edn. Baltimore, MD: Williams & Wilkins, 1994:291–2

Winters RW. Regulation of normal water and electrolyte metabolism. In Winters RW, ed. *The Body Fluids in Pediatrics*, 1st edn. Boston, MA: Little Brown, 1973:99–101

HYPERNATREMIA – FREE WATER DEFICIT

Use

To calculate the free water deficit in hypernatremia (serum sodium > 150 mEq/l).

Formula

$$FWD = \left(\frac{Na - 140}{Na}\right) \times Wt_b \times F \times 1000$$

FWD	=	free water deficit (ml)
Na	=	serum sodium concentration (mEq/l)
Wt_b	=	base line body weight (kg)
F	=	fraction of total body weight that is water

Age	Birth	1 year	Adult male	Adult female
Water fraction of total weight	0.75	0.65	0.60	0.50

Interpretation

This formula estimates free water deficit only when there is no change in total body sodium (e.g. diabetes insipidus) or hypovolemic states when there is disproportionately more water loss than sodium. Therapeutic correction by the administration of hypotonic fluids in dehydrated patients must be undertaken with caution to avoid cerebral edema and neurological complications. The treatment of choice should be aimed at decreasing the serum sodium concentration by no more than 10–12 mEq/day. Therefore, it is safer to set the value of Na in the above formula at 150 mEq/l in dehydrated patients, and to extend the fluid correction over a period of 48 h, while carefully monitoring the serum sodium concentration.

References

Adelman RD, Solhaug MJ. Pathophysiology of body fluids and fluid therapy. In Behrman RE, Kliegman RM, Jenson HB, eds. *Nelson Textbook of Pediatrics*, 16th edn. Philadelphia, PA: WB Saunders, 2000:217

Avner ED. Clinical disorders of water metabolism: hyponatremia and hypernatremia. *Pediatr Ann* 1995;24:23–7

Holliday MA. Fluid and nutrition support. In Holliday MA, Barratt TM, Avner ED, eds. *Pediatric Nephrology*, 3rd edn. Baltimore, MD: Williams & Wilkins, 1994:292

Holliday MA, Segar WE. *Parenteral Fluid Therapy*. Indianapolis, IN: Indiana University Medical Center, 1956:78–80

Winters RW. Regulation of normal water and electrolyte metabolism. In Winters RW, ed. *The Body Fluids in Pediatrics*, 1st edn. Boston, MA: Little Brown, 1973:99–101

CORRECTED SERUM SODIUM – HYPERGLYCEMIA

Use

To calculate the corrected serum sodium concentration in the presence of hyperglycemia.

Formula

$$Na_c = 1.6 \times \left(\frac{G1 - 100}{100} \right) + Na$$

Na_c = corrected serum sodium concentration (mEq/l)
Gl = serum glucose concentration (mg/dl)
Na = measured serum sodium concentration (mEq/l)

Interpretation

Elevated serum glucose will cause an intracellular-to-extracellular shift of water, which reduces the measured serum sodium. In hyperglycemia, therefore, the serum sodium may appear normal when there is hypertonic dehydration with a free water deficit.

References

Adrogue HJ, Madias NE. Hyponatremia. *N Engl J Med* 2000;342:1583

Avner ED. Clinical disorders of water metabolism: hyponatremia and hypernatremia. *Pediatr Ann* 1995;24:26

Hillier TA, Abbot RD, Barrett EJ. Hyponatremia: evaluating the correction factor for hyperglycemia. *Am J Med* 1999;106:399–403

FREE WATER CLEARANCE

Use

To assess whether polyuria (urine volume greater than twice maintenance fluids or > 3000 ml/m^2) represents a water or solute diuresis.

Formula

$$FWC = V \times \left(1 - \frac{Osm_u}{Osm_p}\right)$$

FWC	=	free water clearance (liters/day)
V	=	volume of urine (liters/day)
Osm_u	=	urine osmolality (mOsm/kg H_2O)
Osm_p	=	plasma osmolality (mOsm/kg H_2O)

Interpretation

A positive FWC indicates a water diuresis. A negative FWC indicates a solute diuresis. Additional interpretation, using urine osmolality alone:

Osm_u < 250 mOsm/kg H_2O suggests water diuresis
Osm_u > 300 mOsm/kg H_2O suggests solute diuresis
Osm_u 250–300 mOsm/kg H_2O can occur in mixed water–solute diuresis

References

Haycock GB. Sodium and water. In Holliday MA, Barratt TM, Avner ED, eds. *Pediatric Nephrology*, 3rd edn. Baltimore, MD: Williams & Wilkins, 1994:186

Jamison RL. Urinary concentration and dilution. In Brenner BM, Rector FC Jr, eds. *The Kidney*. Philadelphia, PA: WB Saunders, 1976:394

Oster JR, Singer I, Thatte L, Grant-Taylor I, Diego JM. The polyuria of solute diuresis. *Arch Intern Med* 1997;157:721–9

SERUM POTASSIUM AND ACID–BASE

Use

To determine the effect of acid–base imbalance on serum potassium concentration.

Formulas

Acidosis formula: $\uparrow K_\Delta = \dfrac{AC_F\,(7.4 - pH)}{0.1}$

Alkalosis formula: $\downarrow K_\Delta = \dfrac{AL_F\,(pH - 7.4)}{0.1}$

$\uparrow K_\Delta$	=	increase in serum potassium concentration (mEq/l)
$\downarrow K_\Delta$	=	decrease in serum potassium concentration (mEq/l)
AC_F	=	acidosis factor
AL_F	=	alkalosis factor

Acid–base condition	AC_F and AL_F
Acute mineral acidosis (e.g. acute renal failure)	1.6
Acute organic acidosis (e.g. lactic)	0.0
Acute metabolic alkalosis	0.5
Acute respiratory acidosis	0.7
Acute respiratory alkalosis	0.7
Chronic respiratory acidosis	0.0
Chronic respiratory alkalosis	0.0
Chronic metabolic acidosis	variable

Interpretation

Potassium is displaced extracellularly as hydrogen ions move into the cells in acute mineral metabolic acidosis. This effect is minimal in acute organic acidosis. Changes in pH can cause serum potassium to increase as much as 1.6 mEq/l for every 0.1 unit reduction in arterial pH in severe mineral acidosis. Both acute respiratory acidosis and alkalosis reduce serum potassium concentration, but the change is to a lesser degree than in acidosis. Chronic states of acid–base imbalance cause less change in serum potassium.

References

Adelman RD, Solhaug MJ. Pathophysiology of body fluids and fluid therapy. In Behrman RE, Kleigman RM, Jenson, HB, eds. *Nelson Textbook of Pediatrics*, 16th edn. Philadelphia, PA: WB Saunders, 2000:197

Adrogue HJ, Madias NE. Changes in plasma potassium concentration during acute acid–base disturbances. *Am J Med* 1981;71:456–7

Cogan MG. *Fluid and Electrolytes: Physiology and Pathophysiology.* Norwalk, CT: Appleton & Lange, 1991:107, 160–1

Saxton CR, Seldin DW. Clinical interpretation of laboratory values. In Kokko JP, Tannen RL, eds. *Fluids and Electrolytes.* Philadelphia, PA: WB Saunders, 1986:20

Segel NJ, VanWhy SK, Boydstun II, *et al.* Acute renal failure. In Holliday MA, Barratt TM, Avner ED, eds. *Pediatric Nephrology,* 3rd edn. Baltimore, MD: Williams & Wilkins, 1994:197

TRANSTUBULAR POTASSIUM GRADIENT

Use

To determine whether hyperkalemia is of renal or extrarenal origin.

Formula

$$TTKG = \left(\frac{K_u}{K_s} \times \frac{S_{OSM}}{U_{OSM}} \right)$$

TTKG	=	transtubular potassium gradient
K_u	=	urine potassium (mEq/l)
K_s	=	serum potassium (mEq/)
S_{OSM}	=	serum osmolality (mOsm/kg H_2O)
U_{OSM}	=	urine osmolality (mOsm/kg H_2O)

Interpretation

TTKG > 6 suggests a non-renal cause of hyperkalemia (e.g. increased K intake, hemolysis, rhabdomyolysis, acidosis).

TTKG < 6 suggests a renal cause of hyperkalemia (e.g. aldosterone deficiency or lack of response). In the absence of renal failure, serum aldosterone and renin are helpful for further identification of the cause (see table).

In infants, adrenogenital syndrome with salt wasting is a major cause of aldosterone deficiency.

TTKG	*Serum aldosterone*	*Plasma renin*	*Suggested diagnosis*
> 6			non-renal cause
< 6	low	high	hypoaldosteronism
< 6	low	low	hyporeninemic hypoaldosteronism
< 6	normal	normal	renal tubular defect

Note: Newborns have a low rate of potassium excretion under basal conditions. The validity of using TTKG in infants and children has not been demonstrated.

References

Rastegar A, DeFronzo RA. Disorders of potassium metabolism. In Schrier RW, Gottschalk CE, eds. *Diseases of the Kidney*, 5th edn. Boston, MA: Little Brown, 1993:2658

Satlin LM, Holliday MA. Potasium. In Holliday MA, Barratt TM, Avner ED, eds. *Pediatric Nephrology*, 3rd edn. Baltimore, MD: Williams & Wilkins, 1994:219

TOTAL AND IONIZED SERUM CALCIUM

To convert calcium from mEq/l to mg/dl multiply by 2.
To convert calcium from mmol/l to mg/dl multiply by 4.

Use

To correct total serum calcium concentration for low serum protein.

Formula

$$Ca_c = Ca + [(4 - SA) \times 0.75]$$

Ca_c	=	corrected serum calcium (mg/dl)
Ca	=	total calcium measured (mg/dl)
SA	=	serum albumin (g/dl)

Interpretation

Total serum calcium decreases 0.75 mg/dl per 1.0 g/dl reduction in serum albumin, assuming the normal serum albumin is 4.0 g/dl. With hypoalbuminemia, total serum calcium falls but ionized calcium remains unchanged, and calcium physiology remains normal.

Normal total calcium

Age	Total Ca (mg/dl)
Premature (1st week)	6.0–10.0
Term newborn (1st week)	7.0–12.0
Childhood	8.0–10.5
Adult	8.0–10.5

Ionized serum calcium

Use

To estimate the ionized serum calcium from measured total serum calcium and serum protein.

$$Ca_i = Ca \times \left(1 - \frac{(8 \times SA) + (2 \times Glob) + 3}{100}\right)$$

Ca_i	=	ionized serum calcium (mg/dl)
Ca	=	total measured serum calcium (mg/dl)
SA	=	serum albumin (g/dl)
Glob	=	serum globulin (g/dl)

Interpretation

Normal ionized calcium levels vary in infancy reaching peak levels near 9–14 days of age. Levels are near adult norms after 2 months (see table).

Normal ionized calcium

Age	Ionized calcium (mg/dl)
0–2 days	4.4–5.6
3–4 days	4.4–6.0
5–8 days	4.8–6.0
9–14 days	5.2–6.4
2 months to 18 years	4.8–5.6

Total serum calcium and pH

For alkalosis

$$Ca_c = Ca - \left(\frac{pH - 7.4}{0.1} \times 0.16\right)$$

For acidosis

$$Ca_c = Ca + \left(\frac{7.4 - pH}{0.1} \times 0.16\right)$$

Ca_c	=	corrected serum calcium (mg/dl)
Ca	=	measured serum calcium (mg/dl)
pH	=	measured blood pH

Interpretation

Serum calcium decreases 0.16 mg/dl per 0.1 unit rise in pH (alkalosis), and increases an equal amount in acidosis. In acute pH changes these calcium changes affect both total and ionized calcium, but in more chronic states the ionized calcium returns to normal.

References

Choukair MK. Blood chemistries/body fluids. In Siberry GK, Iannone R, eds. *The Harriet Lane Handbook*, 15th edn. Baltimore, MD: Mosby, 1999:121

Halick MF, Krane SM, Potts JT Jr. Calcium, phosphorus and bone metabolism: calcium regulating hormones. In Isselbacher KJ, Braunwald EW, Wilson JD, *et al*, eds. *Harrison's Principles of Internal Medicine*, 13th edn. New York, NY: McGraw Hill, 1994:2139

Hammond KB. Normal biochemical and hematologic values. In Hay WW Jr, Groothuis JR, Hayward AR, Levin MJ, eds. *Current Pediatric Diagnosis and Treatment*, 13th edn. Stamford, CT: Appleton & Lange, 1997:1127

Portale AA. Calcium and phosphorus. In Holliday MA, Barratt TM, Avner ED, eds. *Pediatric Nephrology*, 3rd edn. Baltimore, MD: Williams & Wilkins, 1994:247

SERUM CALCIUM–PHOSPHORUS CONCENTRATION PRODUCT

Use

To evaluate the risk of soft tissue calcification resulting from elevated calcium and/or phosphorus.

Formula

$CPP = Ca \times P$

CPP	=	serum calcium–phosphorus product
Ca	=	serum calcium measured (mg/dl)
P	=	serum phosphorus (mg/dl)

Interpretation

CPP > 63 suggests risk of soft tissue calcification which may involve the heart, blood vessels, kidneys, lungs and brain.

Reference

Fouser L. Disorders of calcium, phosphorus, and magnesium. *Pediatr Ann* 1995; 24:38

PLASMA OSMOLALITY AND OSMOLAR GAP

Use

To calculate plasma osmolality and osmolar gap.

Plasma osmolality

Formula

$$PO_c = 2 \times Na + \frac{Gl}{18} + \frac{BUN}{2.8}$$

PO_c	=	calculated plasma osmolality (mOsm/kg H_2O)
Na	=	serum sodium concentration (mEq/l)
Gl	=	serum glucose concentration. (mg/dl)
BUN	=	blood urea nitrogen concentration (mg/dl)

Osmolar gap

Formula

$$OG = PO_m - PO_c$$

OG	=	osmolar gap (mOsm/kg H_2O)
PO_m	=	plasma osmolality (mOsm/kg H_2O) measured directly
PO_c	=	calculated plasma osmolality (mOsm/kg H_2O)

Interpretation

Normal $OG = \pm 9$ mOsm/kg H_2O. An increased osmolar gap suggests the presence of a circulating low-molecular weight agent such as ethanol, methanol, ethylene glycol, etc. The increment in osmolar pressure contributed by an exogenous agent can also be estimated by dividing its concentration in mg/dl by its molecular weight and multiplying by 10 (e.g. Δ osmolality = concentration/MW $\times$ 10).

Reference

Cogan MA. *Fluid and Electrolytes: Physiology & Pathophysiology.* Norwalk, CT: Appleton & Lange, 1991:101

OSMOTIC PRESSURE CONTRIBUTED BY EXOGENOUS AGENT

Use

To calculate the osmotic pressure contributed by a known circulating exogenous agent, such as ethanol, methanol, ethylene glycol.

Formula

$$OP = \frac{C_e}{MW} \times 10$$

OP	=	increment in osmotic pressure due to exogenous agent (mOsm/kg H_2O)
C_e	=	concentration of exogenous agent (mg/dl)
MW	=	molecular weight of exogenous agent

Reference

Cogan MA. *Fluid & Electrolytes: Physiology and Pathophysiology.* Norwalk, CT: Appleton & Lange, 1991:101

URINE OSMOLALITY/PLASMA OSMOLALITY RATIO IN POLYURIA

Use

To determine the cause of polyuria.

Formula

$$Ratio = \frac{U_{OSM}}{S_{OSM}}$$

U_{OSM}	=	urine osmolality (mOsm/kg H_2O)
S_{OSM}	=	serum osmolality (mOsm/kg H_2O)

Interpretation

Normal ratio = 1.0–3.0 or higher.
Water intoxication or compulsive water drinking: ratio = < 1.0 (with water deprivation: ratio = > 1.0).
Central diabetes insipidus: ratio = 0.2–0.7 (with water deprivation: ratio = < 1.0; corrects with vasopressin).
Nephrogenic diabetes insipidus: ratio = 0.2–0.7 (with water deprivation: ratio = < 1.0; does not correct with vasopressin).

References

Bacon GE, Spencer ML, Hopwood NJ, Kelch R. *A Practical Approach to Pediatric Endocrinology.* 3rd edn. Chicago, IL: Year Book Medical Publishers, 1990

Brensilver JM, Goldberger E. *A Primer of Water, Electrolyte, and Acid–Base Syndromes*, 8th edn. Philadelphia, PA: FA Davis, 1996:115

Gotlin RW, Kappy MS, Slover RH. Endocrine disorders. In Hay WW Jr, Groothuis JR, Hayward AR, Levin MJ, eds. *Current Pediatric Diagnosis and Treatment*, 13th edn. Stamford, CT: Appleton & Lange, 1997:825

Teitz NW, ed. *Clinical Guide to Laboratory Tests*, 3rd edn. Philadelphia, PA: WB Saunders, 1995:458–9

ENDOCRINE SYSTEM

INSULIN SUPPRESSION TEST

Use

To determine the presence of hyperinsulinemia as a cause of hypoglycemia.

Insulin/glucose ratio formula

$$\text{I : G ratio} = \frac{\text{Ins}}{\text{Gl}}$$

$$\begin{aligned}
\text{Ins} &= \text{serum insulin } (\mu\text{U/ml}) \\
\text{Gl} &= \text{serum glucose (mg/dl)}
\end{aligned}$$

Amended insulin/glucose ratio formula

$$\text{Amended I : G ratio} = \frac{\text{Ins} \times 100}{\text{Gl} - 30}$$

Interpretation

In the presence of hypoglycemia the I : G ratio should be < 0.3, or the amended I : G ratio should be < 30. Higher values would indicate hyperinsulinemic hypoglycemia. In small infants and children the differential considerations include nesidioblastosis, beta cell hyperplasia and beta cell adenoma.

Note: Term neonates are considered hypoglycemic as follows:
Less than 3 h of age: blood glucose < 35 mg/dl
Between 3 and 24 h: blood glucose < 40 mg/dl
More than 24 h: blood glucose < 55 mg/dl

References

Cowett RM. Hypoglycemia in the newborn. In Lifshitz F, ed. *Pediatric Endocrinology*. New York, NY: Marcel Dekker, 1996:677–92
Sperling MA. Hypoglycemia in the infant and child. In Lifshitz F, ed. *Pediatric Endocrinology*. New York, NY: Marcel Dekker, 1996:693–713

SERUM LUTEINIZING HORMONE/FOLLICLE STIMULATING HORMONE RATIO

Use

Diagnosis of polycystic ovary (PCO), Stein–Levinthal syndrome.

Formula

$$\text{LH/FSH ratio} = \frac{\text{LH}}{\text{FSH}}$$

LH	=	serum immunoreactive luteinizing hormone (mIU/ml, IU/l)
FSH	=	serum follicle stimulating hormone (mIU/ml, IU/l)

Interpretation

An LH/FSH ratio greater than 3.5 occurs in 65% of women with PCO syndrome. Because the majority of PCO patients are normogonadotropic, the ratio provides some discriminatory diagnostic information. PCO syndrome is probably a group of closely related syndromes. It is characterized by polycystic ovaries, obesity, hirsutism, anovulation and androgen excess.

References

Lobo RA, Kletzky OA, Campeau JD, diZerega GS. Elevated bioactive luteinizing hormone in women with the polycystic ovary syndrome. *Fertil Steril* 1983;39:674–8
Songya P. Hirsutism and polycystic ovary syndrome. In Lifshitz F, ed. *Pediatric Endocrinology*, 3rd edn. New York, NY: Marcel Dekker, 1996:248

RENAL CALCIUM CLEARANCE/CREATININE CLEARANCE RATIO

Use

To differentiate familial hypocalciuric hypercalcemia from primary hyperparathyroidism.

Formula

$$\text{Ratio} = \frac{\text{Ca}_u}{\text{Ca}} \times \frac{\text{Cr}}{\text{Cr}_u}$$

Ca_u	=	total urine calcium (mg/dl/24 h)
Ca	=	fasting serum calcium (mg/dl)
Cr	=	fasting serum creatinine (mg/dl)
Cr_u	=	urine creatinine (mg/dl/24 h)

Interpretation

A ratio of less than 0.01 suggests familial hypocalciuric hypercalcemia. First-degree relatives should be screened. Familial hypocalciuric hypercalcemia is an autosomal dominant disorder characterized by increased renal tubular reabsorption of filtered calcium. Such patients do not benefit from parathyroidectomy.

References

Aurbach GD, Marx SJ, Dpiegel AM. Parathyroid hormone, calcitonin, and calciferols. In Wilson JD, Foster DW, eds. *Williams Textbook of Endocrinology*, 8th edn. Philadelphia, PA: WB Saunders, 1992:1444

Bainbridge RR, Koo WW, Tsang RC. Neonatal calcium and phosphorus disorders. In Lifshitz F, ed. *Pediatric Endocrinology*, 3rd edn. New York, NY: Marcel Dekker, 1996:486

GASTROINTESTINAL TRACT AND LIVER

SERUM–ASCITES ALBUMIN GRADIENT

Use

To differentiate portal hypertension from non-hepatic pathology as the cause of ascites.

Formula

$SAAG = A - A_{asc}$

SAAG	=	serum–ascites albumin gradient (g/dl)
A	=	serum albumin (g/dl)
A_{asc}	=	ascites albumin (g/l)

Interpretation

SAAG of greater than 1.1 g/dl suggests portal hypertension as the cause of ascites. The following table lists the major causes of ascites secondary to portal hypertension and those without portal hypertension.

Portal hypertension (SAAG > 1.1 g/dl)	No portal hypertension (SAAG < 1.1 g/dl)
Cirrhosis	Neoplastic
Heart failure	Peritoneal tuberculosis
Hepatic failure	Pancreatitis
Hepatic fibrosis (with or without autosomal recessive polycystic kidneys)	Nephrotic syndrome
	Vasculitis (lupus)
Budd–Chiari syndrome	
Veno-occlusive disease (renal vein)	
Neonatal omphalitis	

References

Conn HO, Colin CE. Cirrhosis. In Schiff LS, Schiff ER, eds. *Diseases of the Liver*, 6th edn. Philadelphia, PA: JB Lippincott, 1987:770,886

Runyon BA, Montano AA, Evangelos A, *et al*. The serum–ascites albumin gradient is superior to the exudate–transudate concept in the differential diagnosis of ascites. *Ann Intern Med* 1992;117:215–20

FECAL OSMOTIC GAP

Use

To distinguish between a secretory and an osmotic cause for diarrhea.

Formula

$$FOG = MFO - 2 \times (Na_F + K_F)$$

FOG	=	fecal osmotic gap (mOsm/kg H_2O)
MFO	=	measured fecal osmolality (mOsm/kg H_2O)
Na_F	=	fecal sodium (mEq/l)
K_F	=	fecal potassium (mEq/l)

Interpretation

A fecal osmotic gap of less than 50 mOsm/kg H_2O suggests a secretory mechanism, and a gap greater than 160 mOsm/kg H_2O suggests an osmotic mechanism for the diarrhea. A gap between 50 and 160 suggests a combined mechanism. Alternatively, a stool sodium concentration greater than 70 mEq/l indicates a severe secretory process, and a stool sodium concentration less than 50 mEq/l an osmotic process. Secretory diarrhea occurs with most infectious causes and with phenolphthalein, while osmotic diarrhea is caused either by ingestion of osmotic agents (e.g. $Mg(OH)_2$, lactulose, sorbitol, etc.) or by carbohydrate malabsorption (e.g. lactose intolerance).

Note: Diarrhea is defined as greater than 10 g/kg of stool per day in infants and children, and greater than 200 g per day in adults.

Reference

Riedel BD, Ghishan FK. Acute diarrhea. In Walker WA, Durie PR, Hamilton JR, Walker-Smith JA, Watkins JB, eds. *Pediatric Gastrointestinal Disease*, 2nd edn. St Louis, MO: Mosby-Year Book, 1996:251, 258

HEMATOLOGIC FUNCTION

CORRECTED PERCENT RETICULOCYTE COUNT

Use

To correct the percent reticulocyte count for anemia. Unless corrected, the reticulocyte count (expressed as percent erythrocyte count) will be falsely elevated.

Formula

$$RC_c = RC \times \frac{Hct}{NHct}$$

RC_c	=	corrected reticulocyte count (%)
RC	=	measured reticulocyte count (%)
Hct	=	measured hematocrit (%)
NHct	=	normal hematocrit for age (%)

Interpretation

Normal hematocrit and normal reticulocyte counts

Age	Normal hematocrit	Normal reticulocyte count (%)
28 weeks	41	5–10
32 weeks	44	3–10
Term	51	3–7
1–3 days	56	1.8–4.6
1 month	43	0.1–2.9
6 months	36	0.7–2.3
2–6 years	37	0.5–1.0
6–12 years	40	0.5–1.0
12–18 years	42	0.5–1.0
Adult male	47	0.5–1.5
Adult female	41	0.5–1.5

A corrected reticulocyte count above the normal reticulocyte count for age is considered elevated, and indicates that the bone marrow has increased red cell production. Values that are normal or below the normal reticulocyte count in the presence of anemia indicate that the marrow is not responding.

Note: Hematocrit norms vary with altitude. For persons who live at altitude, add 5% to the listed norms for each 800 m/½ mile elevation.

References

Ebel BE, Raffini L. Hematology. In Siberry GK, Iannone R, eds. *The Harriet Lane Handbook*, 15th edn. Baltimore, MD: Mosby, 1999:325

Nathan DG, Orkin SH, eds. *Nathan and Oski's Hematology of Infancy and Childhood*, 5th edn. Philadelphia, PA: WB Saunders, 1998:31–2,viii

Schwartz E. The anemias. In Behrman RE, Kliegman RM, Jenson HB, eds. *Nelson Textbook of Pediatrics*, 16th edn. Philadelphia, PA: WB Saunders, 2000:1462

ABSOLUTE RETICULOCYTE COUNT

Use

To evaluate the reticulocyte count in the presence of anemia.

Formula

$$ARC = \frac{Retic}{100} \times RBC$$

ARC	=	absolute reticulocyte count (per µl)
Retic	=	reticulocytes reported (%)
RBC	=	measured red blood cell count (per µl)

Interpretation

Normal RBC and absolute reticulocyte counts

Age	RBC × 10^6/µl	Absolute reticulocyte count (per µl) (values are derived and approximate)
28 weeks	4.62	346 500
32 weeks	5.00	325 000
Term	5.14	257 000
1–3 days	5.70	182 400
1 month	4.20	63 000–94 000
6 months	3.80	57 000–85 000
2–6 years	4.60	34 500–50 000
6–12 years	4.60	34 500–50 000
12–18 years	4.60	34 500–75 000
Adult male	5.20	50 000–100 000
Adult female	4.60	50 000–100 000

References

Ebel BE, Raffini L. Hematology. In Siberry GK, Iannone R, eds. *The Harriet Lane Handbook*, 15th edn. Baltimore, MD: Mosby, 1999:325

Nathan DG, Orkin SH, eds. *Nathan and Oski's Hematology of Infancy and Childhood*, 5th edn. Philadelphia, PA: WB Saunders, 1998:31–2,viii

Schwartz E. The anemias. In Behrman RE, Kliegman RM, Jenson HB, eds. *Nelson Textbook of Pediatrics*, 16th edn. Philadelphia, PA: WB Saunders, 2000:1462

PLATELET CORRECTED COUNT INCREMENT

Use

To determine whether platelets transfused for treatment of thrombocytopenia show sufficient survival duration to be therapeutically useful.

Formula

$$CCI = \frac{PostTPC - PreTPC}{PlatT \times 10^{-11}} \times BSA$$

CCI	=	corrected count increment (count/mm^3)
PostTPC	=	post-transfusion platelet count (count/mm^3)
PreTPC	=	pre-transfusion platelet count (count/mm^3)
PlatT	=	total number of platelets transfused (see footnote)*
BSA	=	body surface area (m^2)

Interpretation

15–60 min post-transfusion: CCI of greater than 10 000/mm^3 indicates adequate platelet survival. 18–24 h post-transfusion: CCI of greater than 7500/mm^3 indicates adequate platelet survival.

CCI at 15–60 min	CCI at 24 h	Interpretation
> 10 000	> 7500	adequate platelet survival
> 10 000	< 7500	non-immune process (sepsis, DIC)
< 10 000	< 7500	immune process (alloimmunized, platelet autoantibodies)

DIC, disseminated intravascular coagulation

* In general one unit of random donor platelets contains $5.0–7.0 \times 10^{10}$ platelets, and one unit of single donor platelets contains $3.0–5.0 \times 10^{11}$ platelets. With adequate platelet survival, one random donor unit per 10 kg body weight (or one unit of single donor platelets per 60 kg) should increase the platelet count by 40 000 to 50 000 /mm^3 within 1 h after infusion.

Reference

Nugent DJ. Platelet transfusion. In Nathan DG, Orkin SH, eds. *Nathan and Oski's Hematology of Infancy and Childhood*, 5th edn. Philadelphia, PA: WB Saunders, 1998:1804–6

ERYTHROCYTE INDICES

Use

To evaluate the type and cause of anemia.

Mean corpuscular volume (average red blood cell volume).

Formula

$$MCV = \frac{Hct}{RBC \times 10^{-7}}$$

MCV = mean corpuscular volume (fl = femtoliters = 10^{-15} liters)
Hct = hematocrit (%)
RBC = red blood cell count (per µl)

Interpretation

Normal MCV varies with age in children (see table). An estimate of the lower limit of normal MCV for children from 1 to 8 years can be made by the following formula: Minimum MCV = age in years + 70

MCV norms

Age	MCV mean	MinimumMCV (microcytic)	Maximum MCV (macrocytic)
Birth	108	98	118
1 month	104	86	111
2 months	95	84	106
6 months	84	74	94
1 year	78	70	86
6 years	81	75	86
12 years	86	77	87
18 years	90	80	100

Mean corpuscular hemoglobin (hemoglobin content per RBC)

Formula

$$MCH = \frac{Hb}{RBC \times 10^{-7}}$$

MCH	=	mean corpuscular hemoglobin (pg/cell)
Hb	=	hemoglobin (g/dl)
RBC	=	erythrocyte count (per (μl)

MCH is near 31–37 pg/cell in the 1st month of life, gradually falls to 24–30 pg/cell by 6–24 months, then gradually rises to adult norms of 26–34 pg/cell in adolescence. MCH has no clinical usefulness in infants and children.

Mean corpuscular hemoglobin concentration
(grams of hemoglobin per 100 ml packed RBCs)

Formula

$$MCHC = \frac{Hb}{Hct} \times 100$$

MCHC	=	mean corpuscular hemoglobin concentration (g Hb/dl RBC)
Hb	=	hemoglobin (g/dl)
Hct	=	hematocrit (%)

MCHC varies little with age. Values of 30–36 g/dl are considered normal at all ages. A low, normal, or high MCHC defines hypochromia, normochromia, or hyperchromia, respectively. Hypochromia is seen in iron deficiency and sideroblastic anemias. Hyperchromic anemia is seen in hereditary spherocytosis, sickle cell disease and homozygous hemoglobin C disease.

Red cell distribution width (coefficient of variation in red cell size)

Formula

$$RDW = \frac{SD \text{ of red cell volume}}{MCV} \times 100$$

RDW	=	red cell distribution width
SD of red cell volume	=	a flow cytometric reading of the coefficient of variation of red cell volume of distribution
MCV	=	mean corpuscular volume of red cells

RDW norms remain at 11.5–14.5% for all ages except in the newborn, when values may be higher. RDW is high in anemia of blood loss, hemolytic disease, iron deficiency and disseminated intravascular coagulation (DIC) (see table).

Composite interpretation of erythrocyte indices in anemia

	Mean corpuscular volume (MCV)		
RDW/RETIC	*Low (microcytic)*	*Normal (normocytic)*	*High (macrocytic)*
Normal RDW Low reticulocytes	thalassemia trait lead poisoning aluminum toxicity copper deficiency	anemia of chronic disease anemia of chronic infection acute blood loss endocrinopathies cancer, leukemia chronic renal failure sickle cell trait, Hgb C trait transient erythroblastopenia	aplastic anemia pre-leukemia hypothyroid congenital marrow failure liver disease drug induced folate, B_{12} deficiency trisomy 21
High RDW Low reticulocytes	iron deficiency anemia	early iron deficiency cancer, leukemia	
High RDW High reticulocytes	thalassemia (homozygous) anemia of chronic disease chronic blood loss	sickle cell, Hgb C disease microangiopathic hemolytic anemia (DIC) hypersplenism congenital spherocytosis RBC membrane and enzyme disorders	newborn hemolytic disease immune hemolytic disease

References

Ebel BE, Raffini L. Hematology. In Siberry GK, Iannone R, eds. *The Harriet Lane Handbook*, 15th edn. Baltimore, MD: Mosby, 1999:307–10
Evans TC, Jehle D. The red blood cell distribution width. *J Emerg Med* 1991;9:71–4
Nathan DG, Orkin SH, eds. *Nathan and Oski's Hematology of Infancy and Childhood*, 5th edn. Philadelphia, PA: WB Saunders, 1998:31–2, iii–vi

TRANSFERRIN SATURATION

Use

To evaluate the status of iron storage.

Formula

$$\% \text{ Saturation} = \frac{\text{SI}}{\text{TIBC}} \times 100$$

% Saturation	=	percent maximum saturation of transferrin with iron
SI	=	serum iron (μg/dl)
TIBC	=	total iron binding capacity (μg/dl)

Interpretation

Normal transferrin saturation varies somewhat with age.

Normal range of transferrin saturation

Age	% Transferrin saturation
1–5 years	16–28
6–9 years	23–36
10–14 years	11–30
14–19 ycars	12–27

Generally, transferrin saturations below these percentages suggest iron deficiency. In children with renal failure, transferrin saturation should be maintained above 20% with iron supplementation. Above 50% is consistent with iron overload (hemochromatosis, hemosiderosis, iron poisoning).

References

Fairbanks VF, Baldus WP. Iron overload (hemochromatosis). In Bennet JC, Plum F, eds. *Cecil Textbook of Medicine*, 20th edn. Philadelphia, PA: WB Saunders, 1996:1132–5

Harmon WE, Jabs K. Hemodialysis. In Holliday MA, Barratt TM, Avner ED, eds. *Pediatric Nephrology*, 3rd edn. Baltimore, MD: Williams & Wilkins, 1994:1364

Nathan DG, Orkin SH, eds. *Nathan and Oski's Hematology of Infancy and Childhood*, 5th edn. Philadelphia, PA: WB Saunders, 1998:xxii

TOTAL IRON DEFICIENCY

Use

To estimate the total iron deficiency in iron deficiency anemia.

Formula

TFe = [2.21 × Wt × (NHb − MHb)] + (13 × Wt)

TFe   =   total body iron deficiency (mg)
Wt   =   ideal body weight (kg)
NHb   =   normal hemoglobin for age (g/dl)
MHb   =   measured hemoglobin (g/dl)

Age	Mean normal hemoglobin (g/dl)
Birth	16.5
1 week	17.5
1 month	14.0
3–6 months	11.5
6 months to 2 years	12.0
2–6 years	13.5
12–18 years	14.0–14.5

Interpretation

The above formula estimates the total body iron deficiency in milligrams.
For the intravenous dosing with iron dextran (50 mg of elemental iron per ml)
use the following formula:

$$ID = [0.0442 \times Wt \times (NHb - MHb)] + (0.26 \times Wt) \quad (\text{Maximum dose is 14 ml})$$

ID   =   iron dextran (total ml)

The formula yields only an approximation of the amount of iron required in
the individual patient for repletion intravenously. The formula cannot be used
for oral therapy because of the low and variable iron absorption from the gastrointestinal tract.

References

Andrews NC, Bridges KR. Disorders of iron metabolism and sideroblastic anemia. In
Nathan DG, Orkin SH, eds. *Nathan and Oski's Hematology of Infancy and
Childhood*, 5th edn. Philadelphia, PA: WB Saunders, 1998:442, viii
Siberry GK, Iannone R, eds. *The Harriet Lane Handbook*, 15th edn. Baltimore, MD:
Mosby, 1999:743

RBC TRANSFUSION VOLUME

Use

To estimate the total volume of packed RBCs to transfuse.

Formula

$$RBC_v = EBV \times Wt \times \frac{Hct_d - Hct_a}{Hct_t}$$

RBC$_v$	=	volume of packed RBCs to transfuse (ml)
EBV	=	estimated blood volume of patient (ml/kg) (see table)
Wt	=	weight (kg)
Hct$_d$	=	hematocrit desired (%)
Hct$_a$	=	patient's actual hematocrit (%)
Hct$_t$	=	hematocrit of transfused RBCs (usually 55–70%)

Interpretation

In severely anemic children, this total RBC volume should be tranfused in small aliquots, each aliquot over 2–4 h. A safe aliquot volume = hemoglobin (g/dl) × kg.

Approximate blood volumes

Age	Blood volume (ml/kg)
Preterm	95
Term newborn	82
1–12 months	78
1–3 years	74
4–6 years	80
7–18 years	88
Adults	68–88

References

Ebel BE, Raffini L. Hematology. In Siberry GK, Iannone R, eds. *The Harriet Lane Handbook*, 15th edn. Baltimore, MD: Mosby, 1999:319
Nathan DG, Orkin SH, eds. *Nathan and Oski's Hematology of Infancy and Childhood*, 5th edn. Philadelphia, PA: WB Saunders, 1998:xiv

PARTIAL EXCHANGE TRANSFUSION

Use

To calculate the volume of packed RBCs needed for a 'double volume' exchange.

Formula

$$RBC_v = EBV \times Wt \times \frac{Hct_a \times 2}{Hct_t}$$

RBC_v	=	volume of packed RBCs to transfuse (ml)
EBV	=	estimated blood volume of patient (ml/kg) (see table)
Wt	=	weight (kg)
Hct_a	=	patient's actual hematocrit (%)
Hct_t	=	hematocrit of transfused RBCs (usually 55–70%)

Interpretation

The formula gives the total volume of packed RBCs to use for a double volume exchange transfusion. This may be indicated in sickle cell patients with acute chest syndrome, stroke, pain crisis or priapism.

Approximate blood volumes

Age	Blood volume (ml/kg)
Preterm	95
Term newborn	82
1–12 months	78
1–3 years	74
4–6 years	80
7–18 years	88
Adults	68–88

References

Ebel BE, Raffini L. Hematology. In Siberry GK, Iannone R, eds. *The Harriet Lane Handbook*, 15th edn. Baltimore, MD: Mosby, 1999:321

Nathan DG, Orkin SH, eds. *Nathan and Oski's Hematology of Infancy and Childhood*, 5th edn. Philadelphia, PA: WB Saunders, 1998:xiv

INFECTIOUS DISEASE

CATHETER-RELATED BACTEREMIA

Use

To determine whether a bacteremia is caused by an infected indwelling venous catheter.

Formula

$$R = \frac{C_{CC}}{V_{CC}}$$

R	=	ratio
C_{CC}	=	catheter bacterial colony count (colonies/ml)
V_{CC}	=	venous bacterial colony count (colonies/ml)

Interpretation

A ratio of quantitative colony counts from blood sampled from a deep catheter to peripheral blood greater than 5 suggests that the bacteremia is secondary to an internally infected deep catheter.

References

Giner M, Meguid MM, Mosca R, Forbes B. The bacteriologic diagnosis of catheter related sepsis. The advantages of quantitative blood cultures. *Nutr Hosp* 1989;4:43–7

Mosca R, Curtas S, Forbes B, Meguid MM. The benefits of isolator cultures in the management of suspected catheter sepsis. *Surgery* 1987;102:718–23

Salzman MB, Rubin LG. Intravenous catheter-related infections. *Adv Pediatr Infect Dis* 1995;10:337–68

CEREBROSPINAL FLUID/SERUM ANTIBODY INDEX

Use

To determine whether antibody present in the cerebrospinal fluid (CSF) was produced in the central nervous system (CNS) or was produced systemically and transported hematogenously into the CNS.

Formula

$$CSF : SAI = \frac{CSFVIgG}{CSFIgG} \times \frac{SIgG}{SVIgG}$$

CSF : SAI	=	CSF : serum antibody index
CSFVIgG	=	spinal fluid antiviral IgG (mg%)*
CSFIgG	=	spinal fluid total IgG (mg%)
SIgG	=	serum total IgG (mg%)
SVIgG	=	serum antiviral IgG (mg%)*

*These two measurements may be expressed as decimal titers (e.g. 0.05 for titer of 1 : 20), as long as both are expressed in the same units.

Interpretation

A CSF : SAI ≥ 1.5 suggests that the antibody was produced within the CNS, indicating that an infection in the CNS is present.

Reference

Tyler KL. Aseptic meningitis, viral encephalitis, and prion diseases. In Fauci AS, Braunwald E, Isselbacher KJ, *et al.*, eds. *Harrison's Principles of Internal Medicine*, 14th edn. New York, NY: McGraw Hill, 1998:2440–1

METABOLISM

QUANTITATIVE BLOOD LIPIDS

Use

To estimate the low-density lipoprotein cholesterol concentration.

Formula

$$LDL = Chol - HDL - \frac{Tg}{5}$$

LDL	=	low-density lipoprotein cholesterol (mg/dl)
Chol	=	total cholesterol (mg/dl)
HDL	=	high-density lipoprotein cholesterol (mg/dl)
Tg	=	triglyceride (mg/dl)

Note: Tg/5 is an estimate of very-low-density lipoprotein cholesterol, and is valid only when the triglyceride is less than 400 mg/dl.

Interpretation in children

Plasma content (mg/dl)	Desirable	Borderline	Undesirable
Total cholesterol	< 170	170–200	> 200
LDL	< 110	110–130	> 130
HDL	> 40	35–40	< 35
Triglyceride	< 70–100	100–125	> 125

The American Heart Association and the American Academy of Pediatrics Committee on Nutrition recommend dietary treatment for hypercholesterolemia (LDL > 110 mg/dl) in children older than 2 years with (1) no more than 30% of total calories as fat, equally distributed among saturated, monounsaturated, and polyunsaturated fats; (2) no more than 100 mg of cholesterol/100 calories (maximum 300 mg/24 h); and (3) the lower limit of fat intake 20% of total calories. Such restrictions under 2 years of age may lead to growth restriction.

Reference

Tershakovec AM, Rader DJ. Disorders of lipoprotein metabolism and transport. In Behrman RE, Kliegman RM, Jenson HB, eds. *Nelson Textbook of Pediatrics*, 16th edn. Philadelphia, PA: WB Saunders, 2000:389–90

LACTATE/PYRUVATE RATIO

Use

To define the type of metabolic defect present in cases of lactic acidosis.

Formula

$$\text{Ratio} = \frac{L}{P}$$

L	=	arterial L(+) lactate (mEq/l)
P	=	arterial L(−) pyruvate (mEq/l)

Interpretation

Normal lactate	=	< 1.5 mEq/l
Normal pyruvate	=	< 0.15 mEq/l
Normal L/P ratio	=	< 10

Glucose is metabolized via the glycolytic cycle to pyruvate, which is then oxidized through the tricarboxylic cycle to CO_2 and H_2O. Normally a minor fraction of the pyruvate is reduced by the pyruvate dehydrogenase enzyme complex to lactate. When this latter metabolic process is excessive, lactic acidosis occurs. Lactic acidosis can be suspected when there is an elevated anion gap with a negative serum Acetest.

Lactic acidosis is of two types. Type A is an anaerobic defect resulting from an insufficient O_2 supply to meet tissue demands. It is characterized by a normal pyruvate, elevated L/P ratio and elevated NADH/NAD ratio. This can be caused by hypoxic states and defects in the respiratory chain of metabolism. Type B is an aerobic defect resulting from a variety of metabolic abnormalities, and is characterized by an elevated pyruvate, normal L/P ratio and normal NADH/NAD ratio. Examples of the latter include genetic defects in fatty acid oxidation, organic acidosis and biotin utilization. These conditions may be identified by specific urinary organic acids and an increase in plasma acylcarnitine profile.

Type A: increased L/P ratio, normal pyruvate	Type B: normal L/P ratio, increased pyruvate	
Normal urine organic acids *Normal plasma acylcarnitine*	*Abnormal urine organic acids* *Elevated plasma acylcarnitine*	*Normal urine organic acids* *Normal plasma acylcarnitine*

Tissue hypoxia
Respiratory chain
	Hypoglycemia
	  fatty acid oxidation
	
	Organic acidosis
	  propionic
	  methylmalonic
	  other
	
	Skin rash/alopecia
	  biotinidase
	  holocarboxylase
	  synthetase
		Hypoglycemia
		  glycogen storage, type 1
		  fatty acid oxidation
		  defects
		  fructose 1,6-, diphosphatase
		  phosphoenolpyruvate
		  carboxykinase
		
		Hyperglycemia
		  diabetes mellitus
		
		Normoglycemia
		  pyruvate dehydrogenase
		  pyruvate carboxylase

Reference

Tershakovec AM, Rader DJ. Defects in intermediary carbohydrate metabolism associated with lactic acidosis. In Behrman RE, Kliegman RM, Jenson HB, eds. *Nelson Textbook of Pediatrics*, 16th edn. Philadelphia, PA: WB Saunders, 2000:414–17

NUTRITION

CALORIC EXPENDITURE

Use

To estimate the maintenance calories expended (and caloric needs) for an average hospitalized infant or child.

Pediatric formulas

For body weight 0–10 kg

$Kcal = Wt \times 100$

For body weight 10–20 kg

$Kcal = 1000 + [(Wt - 10) \times 50]$

For body weight > 20 kg

$Kcal = 1500 + [(Wt - 20) \times 20]$

$$Kcal = \text{kilocalories/24 h}$$
$$Wt = \text{body weight (kg)}$$

Interpretation

The estimation of calories expended forms the basis of determining the maintenance caloric needs for hospitalized infants and children. It also forms the basis of determining the maintenance fluid requirements. The number of calories expended is equal to the number of milliliters of fluid required to replace the average urinary and insensible water losses minus preformed water.

In growing children, of the total calories expended, about 50% are for basic metabolic needs, 12% for growth, 25% for physical activity, 8% for fecal loss and 5% for the thermal effect of food metabolism.

Caloric requirements must be adjusted for activity and ideal weight. The following table shows the caloric needs from the basal state to high activity. The attached figure gives a graphic display of the same information.

Weight (kg)	Basal (Kcal/24 h)	Above formulas	High activity (Kcal/24 h)
10	500	1000	1250
20	800	1500	2000
30	1100	1700	2500
50	1500	2100	3000
70	1700	2500	3300

For adults, resting metabolic rate (RMR) varies with sex and can be estimated by the following.

Adult formulas

Males: $RMR(Kcal/24\ h) = 900 + (10 \times Wt)$
Females: $RMR(Kcal/24\ h) = 800 + (7 \times Wt)$

Activity factor adjustment:

Low: $1.2 \times RMR$
Medium: $1.4 \times RMR$
High: $1.6 \times RMR$

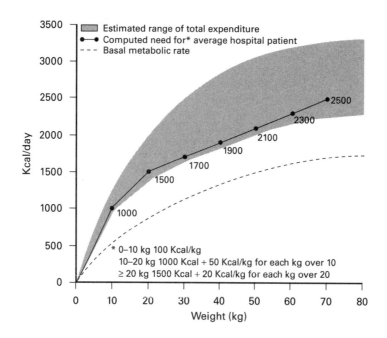

66

References

Harris JA, Benedict FG. A biometric study of basal metabolism in man. In *Carnegie Institution Publication No 279*. Washington, DC: Carnegie Institution, 1919

Holliday MA, Segar WE. *Parenteral Fluid Therapy*. Indianapolis, IN: Indiana University Medical Center, 1956:3–4

Holliday MA, Segar WE. The maintenance need for water in parenteral fluid therapy. *Pediatrics* 1957;19:823–32

Holliday MA. Fluid and nutrition support. In Holliday MA, Barratt TM, Avner ED, eds. *Pediatric Nephrology*, 3rd edn. Baltimore, MD: Williams & Wilkins, 1994:287–9

Pi-Sunyer FX. Obesity. In Bennet JC, Plum F, eds. *Cecil Textbook of Medicine*, 20th edn. Philadelphia, PA: WB Saunders, 1996:1161

PROTEIN REQUIREMENT

Use

To estimate the recommended protein allowance in infants and children.

Formula 1

$$PA = 1.25 \times \left\{ \frac{6.25}{1000} \times \left[\left(\frac{1.5 \times NI}{0.7} \right) + MN \right] \right\} = 0.01674\ NI + 0.00781\ MN$$

or

Formula 2

$$PA = 1.25 \times [(0.01339 \times NI) + (0.00625 \times MN)]$$

$$
\begin{aligned}
PA &= \text{protein allowance (g/kg/day)} \\
NI &= \text{nitrogen increment for growth (mg/kg/day)} \\
MN &= \text{maintenance nitrogen (mg/kg/day)}
\end{aligned}
$$

Interpretation

The formula to determine the protein requirements in infants and children must account for both growth and maintenance needs. Both of these vary with age (see table). Formula 1 above identifies the elements. Growth requirements are multiplied by 1.5 to allow for variability in growth rate, and protein efficiency is estimated at 70%. Protein is considered to contain 16% nitrogen, thus the factor of 6.25/1000 converting milligrams of nitrogen to grams of protein. The coefficient of variation was estimated at 12.5%, so 25% was added to the final equations. Formula 1 can be reduced to Formula 2.

The following table lists the nitrogen requirements for both growth and maintenance.

Age	Nitrogen increment for growth (NI) (mg/kg/day)	Maintenance nitrogen (MN) (mg/kg/day)
3–6 months	47	120
6–12 months	34	120
1 year	16	119
5 years	9	116
9 years	8	111
Males		
12 years	9	108
17 years	3	103
Females		
12 years	7	108
17 years	0	103

References

Hambridge KM, Krebs NF. Normal childhood nutrition and its disorders. In Hay WW Jr, Groothuis JR, Hayward AR, Levin MJ, eds. *Current Pediatric Diagnosis and Treatment*, 13th edn. Stamford, CT: Appleton & Lange, 1997:260

Tershakovec AM, Rader DJ. Defects in intermediary carbohydrate metabolism associated with lactic acidosis. In Behrman RE, Kliegman RM, Jenson HB, eds. *Nelson Textbook of Pediatrics*, 16th edn. Philadelphia, PA: WB Saunders, 2000:414–17

Wassner SJ. Protein and energy. In Holliday MA, Barratt TM, Avner ED, eds. *Pediatric Nephrology*, 3rd edn. Baltimore, MD: Williams & Wilkins; 1994:166–9

NITROGEN BALANCE

Use

To assess the adequacy of protein intake.

Formulas

$$NB = \frac{PI}{6.25} - \left[\frac{UUN}{0.8} + \frac{0.1 \times PI}{6.25} + (0.0075 \times Wt) + \frac{(NI \times Wt)}{1000} \right]$$

which reduces to

$$NB = 0.144 \, PI - \left[1.25 \, UUN + Wt \left(\frac{NI}{1000} + 0.0075 \right) \right]$$

NB = nitrogen balance (g/day)
PI = protein intake (g/day)

UUN = urine urea nitrogen (g/day)

NI = nitrogen increment for growth (mg/kg/day) – see table below

Wt = body weight (kg)

Interpretation

The NB should be a positive value. The above formula makes several assumptions: (1) 6.25 converts grams of protein to grams of nitrogen (proteins average 16% nitrogen); (2) urine nitrogen is 80% urea nitrogen; (3) protein digestibility is 90% (10% lost in stool); (4) integumental nitrogen loss is 7.5 mg/kg/day; (5) there is a certain amount of ingested nitrogen which is retained for growth; and (6) there is no significant change in blood urea nitrogen concentration or body weight, nor is there any significant body fluid drainage during the balance study.

The following table lists the nitrogen requirements for growth.

Age	*Nitrogen increment for growth (NI)* *(mg/kg/day)*
3–6 months	47
6–12 months	34
1 year	16
5 years	9
9 years	8
Males	
12 years	9
17 years	3
Females	
12 years	7
17 years	0

References

Hambridge KM, Krebs NF. Normal childhood nutrition and its disorders. In Hay WW Jr, Groothuis JR, Hayward AR, Levin MJ, eds. *Current Pediatric Diagnosis and Treatment*, 13th edn. Stamford, CT: Appleton & Lange, 1997:260

Heymsfield SB, Williams PJ. Nutritional assessment by anthropometric and biochemical methods. In Shils ME, Olson JA, Shike M, eds. *Modern Nutrition in Health and Disease*, 8th edn. Philadelphia, PA: Lea & Febiger, 1994:829–34

Wassner SJ. Protein and energy. In Holliday MA, Barratt TM, Avner ED, eds. *Pediatric Nephrology*, 3rd edn. Baltimore, MD: Williams & Wilkins, 1994: 166–9

DIETARY PROTEIN INTAKE

Use

To estimate the daily dietary intake of protein from 24 h urea nitrogen excretion, assuming there is a normal anabolic state.

Formula

$$DPI = \left[\left(1.25 \, UUN - \frac{NI \times Wt}{1000} \right) \times 6.25 \right] + P_u$$

DPI	=	dietary protein intake (g/day)
UUN	=	urine urea nitrogen (g/day)
NI	=	nitrogen increment for growth (mg/kg/day) – see table below
Wt	=	body weight (kg)
P_u	=	urine protein (g/day)

Interpretation

The above formula assumes that 80% of urine nitrogen is present in urea, and that a significant amount of ingested nitrogen is retained for growth.

The following table lists the nitrogen requirements for growth.

Age	Nitrogen increment for growth (NI) (mg/kg/day)
3–6 months	47
6–12 months	34
1 year	16
5 years	9
9 years	8
Males	
12 years	9
17 years	3
Females	
12 years	7
17 years	0

References

Hambridge KM, Krebs NF. Normal childhood nutrition and its disorders. In Hay WW Jr, Groothuis JR, Hayward AR, Levin MJ, eds. *Current Pediatric Diagnosis and Treatment*, 13th edn. Stamford, CT: Appleton & Lange, 1997:260

Heymsfield SB, Williams PJ. Nutritional assessment by anthropometric and biochemical methods. In Shils ME, Olson JA, Shike M, eds. *Modern Nutrition in Health and Disease*, 8th edn. Philadelphia, PA: Lea & Febiger, 1994:829–34

Robinson CR, Lawler MR, Chenoweth WL, Garwick AE. *Normal and Therapeutic Nutrition*, 17th edn. New York, NY: Macmillan, 1986:57

Wassner SJ. Protein and energy. In Holliday MA, Barratt TM, Avner ED, eds. *Pediatric Nephrology*, 3rd edn. Baltimore, MD: Williams & Wilkins, 1994:166–9

CALORIC REQUIREMENT OF BURN PATIENTS

Use

To calculate daily caloric requirements of burn patients according to the extent of injury.

Formula

$$\text{Cal} = (\text{BSA} \times 1000) + \left(\text{BSB} \times 40 \times \frac{\text{BSA}}{1.73} \right)$$

BSA	=	body surface area (m^2)
Cal	=	total daily caloric requirement (kcal)
BSB	=	body surface burned (%)

Interpretation

The formula estimates the basal metabolic need at 1000 kcal/m^2. Severely burned patients require more than the usual maintenance energy. This additional energy is proportional to the extent of the burn and the size of the patient. For an adult (1.73 m^2) this additional energy is estimated at 40 kcal per 1% burn.

Percent of body surface area

The 'rule of nines' used in adults can be used only in patients over 14 years. For estimation of surface area (%) in children, the following table can be used.

	Newborn	*3 years*	*6 years*	*12 years*	*Adult*
Head and neck	18	15	12	10	9
Trunk	40	40	40	38	36
Arms	16	16	16	18	18
Legs	26	29	32	34	36

References

Antoon AY, Donovan MK. Burn injuries. In Behrman RE, Kliegman RM, Jenson HB, eds. *Nelson Textbook of Pediatrics*, 16th edn. Philadelphia, PA: WB Saunders, 2000:289–91

Curreri PW. Dietary requirements of patients with major burns. *J Am Diet Assoc* 1974;65:415

Moylan JA. Burn injury. In Carlson RW, Gehab MA, eds. *Principles and Practice of Medical Intensive Care*. Philadelphia, PA: WB Saunders, 1993:1624

ENERGY REQUIREMENTS

Use

To estimate energy requirements in children.

Formula

$E_t = REE \times (1 + F_s) \times Wt_i$

where: REE = 55 − 2A

E_t	=	total daily energy requirement (kcal/day)
REE	=	resting energy expenditure (kcal/kg/day)
F_s	=	sum of factors (fraction added) – see table
Wt_i	=	ideal body weight (kg)
A	=	age (years)

Final formula

$E_t = [55 − 2A] \times (1 + F_s) \times Wt_i$

Interpretation

This formula gives reasonably close estimates of energy needs in children 1–15 years of age. For infants under 1 year, REE = 53–56 kcal/kg/day, and for adult males and females, REE is 27 and 25 kcal/kg/day, respectively.

Adjustments for	Incremental factors (fractions)
Maintenance	0.20
Activity	0.10–0.25
Fever (per degree over 38°C)	0.13
Growth	0.50

Note: Trauma and burns would also increase the overall energy requirements.

References

Cox J. Nutrition: estimating energy needs. In Siberry GK, Iannone R, eds. *The Harriet Lane Handbook*, 15th edn. Baltimore, MD: Mosby, 2000:483–4

Curran JS, Barness LA. Nutrition. In Behrman RE, Kleigman RM, Jenson, HB, eds. *Nelson Textbook of Pediatrics*, 16th edn. Philadelphia, PA: WB Saunders, 2000:138–42

Food Nutrition Board, National Research Council. *Recommended Dietary Allowances*, 10th edn. Washington, DC: National Academy Press, 1989:24–38

Seashore JH. Nutritional support of children in the intensive care unit. *Yale J Biol Med* 1984;57:111–32

PHARMACOKINETICS

LOADING DOSE

Use

To calculate the single loading dose to initiate therapy for a particular drug.

Formula

$$LD = Vd \times Wt \times C_p$$

LD	=	loading dose (mg)
Vd	=	volume of distribution (liters/kg)
Wt	=	body weight (kg)
C_p	=	desired plasma drug concentration (µg/ml)

Volume of distribution is obtained from the Product Information section of the Physician's Desk Reference (PDR) or the package information that accompanies the drug. It is usually described under the heading of Clinical Pharmacology. If actual weight is not available, ideal body weight can be derived from the formulas in the section 'Ideal body weight and height in children', or by consulting standard growth charts (see reference below). Unfortunately, volume of distribution may vary considerably with age and body size.

References

CDC Growth Charts. Bethesda, MD: National Center for Chronic Disease Prevention and Health Promotion, November 21, 2000 (revised and corrected)

Wong AF, Bounger AM, Gambertoglio JG. Pharmacokinetics and drug dosing in children with decreased renal function. In Holliday MA, Barratt TM, Avner ED, eds. Pediatric Nephrology, 3rd edn. Baltimore, MD: Williams & Wilkins, 1994:1306

DIGOXIN OVERDOSE

Use

To calculate the dose of digoxin-specific Fab fragments in a digoxin overdose.

Formula 1 – acute ingestion

$$DIF = \frac{D \times 0.8 \times 38}{0.5}$$

DIF   =   digoxin-specific Fab fragments (mg)
D   =   dose of digoxin ingested (mg)

Interpretation

This formula assumes 80% absorption, and that 38 mg of DIF will bind 0.5 mg of digoxin. Each vial of DIF contains 38 mg of antigen-binding fragments.

Formula 2 – chronic ingestion in children

$$DIF = \frac{DL_s \times Wt \times 38}{100}$$

DIF   =   digoxin-specific Fab fragments (mg)
DL_S =   digoxin serum level (ng/ml)
Wt   =   body weight (kg)

Interpretation

This formula is based on the serum digoxin level in ng/ml. The 38-mg vial of DIF will have to be diluted with saline to facilitate administering the small dose in infants and children.

Reference

Physician's Desk Reference, 55th edn. Montvale, NJ: Medical Economics, 2001:1372–3

INTRAVENOUS DRUG INFUSION

Use

To determine the amount of drug (mg) to be added to 100 ml of fluid to provide a dosing of 1 µg/kg/min, at a rate of 1 ml/h.

Formula

$$MG_{100} = 6 \times Wt$$

MG_{100} =   amount of drug to be added to 100 ml of IV fluid (mg)
Wt   =   body weight (kg)

Interpretation

The formula provides a convenient starting concentration of drug per 100 ml of IV fluid to provide 1 µg/kg/min at a constant infusion rate of 1 ml/h.

Example: Weight 20 kg, desired drug infusion rate of 1 µg/kg/min.

$$MG_{100} \quad = \quad 6 \times 20 = 120 \text{ mg}$$

Thus, adding 120 mg to 100 ml of fluid running at 1 ml/h will provide 1 µg/kg/min.

Reference

Siberry GK, Iannone R, eds. *The Harriet Lane Handbook*, 15th edn. Baltimore, MD: Mosby, 1999

DIGOXIN DOSING IN RENAL FAILURE

Use

To assist in adjusting maintenance digoxin dosing in pediatric patients with reduced renal function.

Formula

$$MD = \frac{\%DL}{100} \times TBC$$

MD	=	maintenance dose (µg/kg/day)
%DL	=	percent digitalizing dose lost daily
TBC	=	total body content (µg/kg)

Interpretation

For practical purposes, the TBC can be equal to the total digitalizing dose, and the %DL is 37% in normal adults, of which 23% is renal and 14% is biliary (creatinine clearance 115 ml/min/1.73 m^2). In infants and children, daily losses are closer to 15% and 10%, respectively.

In infants and children digitalizing doses are larger based on body size because of a larger volume of distribution, and because there is some renal tubular secretion. The volume of distribution of digoxin is 7.5 l/kg in neonates, 16 l/kg in infants and children, and 4 l/kg in adults.

Accordingly, the following formulas can be used to approximate the %DL in adults and children with renal impairment:

Adults:

$$\%DL = 14 + \frac{C_{CR}}{5}$$

Infants and children:

$$\%DL = 10 + \frac{C_{CR}}{7.5}$$

$$C_{CR} = \text{creatinine clearance (ml/min/1.73m}^2)$$

The following table provides the starting digoxin doses for total digitalization, and maintenance, based on normal kidney function and 25% daily loss.

Age	Total digitalizing dose* (µg/kg)	Maintenace (µg/kg/day)
Prematures	20	5
Newborns	30	8
Under 2 years	40–50	10–12
Over 2 years	30–40	8–10

*Note: Digitalizing dose in severe renal impairment should be 50% of the dose listed. Method of digitalizing is not included here.

Another, perhaps more practical, approach to the pediatric patient with renal impairment is to estimate 'percent normal GFR' described elsewhere, and adjust the maintenance dosage based on the following table:

Method of adjustment	> 50% GFR	10–50% GFR	< 10% GFR
% of usual dose given daily	100	50	10
Interval change of usual dose (h)	q 24	q 36	q 48

References

Bresnahan JF. General pharmacology: digoxin. In Brandenburg RO, Fuster V, Giuliani ER, McGoon DC, eds. *Cardiology: Fundamentals and Practice.* Chicago, IL: Year Book Publishers, 1987:531–7

Jelliffe RW. Administration of digoxin. *Dis Chest* 1969;56:58–9

Park MK. *Pediatric Cardiology for Practitioners*, 3rd edn. St Louis, MO: Mosby, 1996:405–6

Smith TW. Heart failure. In Bennett JC, Plum F, eds. *Cecil Textbook of Medicine*, 20th edn. Philadelphia, PA: WB Saunders, 1996:226

PULMONARY FUNCTION

ALVEOLAR–ARTERIAL OXYGEN GRADIENT

Use

To determine whether hypoxemia is due to pulmonary disease or hypoventilation.

Formula

$$AaOG = PAO_2 - PaO_2$$

where:

$$PAO_2 = [FIO_2 \times (P_b - PH_2O)] - \frac{PaCO_2}{R}$$

Simplified formula (assuming breathing room air at sea level when R = 0.8)

$$AaOG = 149 - \frac{PaCO_2}{0.8} - PaO_2$$

AaOG	=	alveolar–arterial oxygen gradient (mmHg)
PAO_2	=	alveolar oxygen pressure (mmHg)
PaO_2	=	measured arterial oxygen pressure (mmHg)
FIO_2	=	fractional O_2 content of inspired gas (0.209 for room air at sea level)
P_b	=	barometric pressure (mmHg) (760 at sea level)
PH_2O	=	water vapor pressure (mmHg) (47 at 37° C)
$PaCO_2$	=	arterial CO_2 tension (mmHg)
R	=	respiratory quotient = ratio of CO_2 produced to O_2 consumed (assumed to be 0.8)

Interpretation

The approximate PAO_2 and PaO_2 at sea level in room air are 100 mmHg and 95 mmHg, respectively. The normal AaOG is therefore near 5 mmHg. However, the AaOG differs somewhat with age and may reach 10 mmHg in a

78

20-year-old, and as high as 20 mmHg in a 65-year-old, because of airway closure and lower ventilation/perfusion ratios in the lung bases in older individuals. Higher AaOG values are seen with diffusion impairment, shunts and ventilation/perfusion mismatching. AaOG remains normal when hypoxemia and CO_2 retention are caused by hypoventilation (depressed respiratory drive, neuromuscular disease).

References

Moylan JA. Burn injury. In Carlson RW, Gehab MA, eds. *Principles and Practice of Medical Intensive Care*. Philadelphia, PA: WB Saunders, 1993:744

O'Brodovich HM, Haddad GG. The functional basis of respiratory pathology. In Chernick V, Kendig EL Jr, eds. *Kendig's Disorders of the Respiratory Tract in Children*, 5th edn. Philadelphia, PA: WB Saunders, 1990:27–8

Yorgin PD, Rhee KH. Gas exchange and acid–base physiology. In Taussig LM, Landau LI, eds. *Pediatric Respiratory Medicine*. St Louis, MO: Mosby, 1999:213

FEV$_1$/FVC RATIO

Use

To differentiate obstructive from restrictive lung disease.

Formula

$$\text{Ratio} = \frac{\text{FEV}_1}{\text{FVC}}$$

$$
\begin{aligned}
\text{FEV}_1 &= \text{forced expiratory volume in 1 s (liters)} \\
\text{FVC} &= \text{forced vital capacity (liters)}
\end{aligned}
$$

Interpretation

Normal ratio in children is 0.86 ± 0.07 (1 SD). In patients with lung disease, lower values indicate obstructive lung disease, and normal or higher values indicate restrictive lung disease.

Note: Measurement of FVC in children may be unreliable before the age of 6 years. Criteria for accepting results in children include: (1) appropriate curve shape; (2) artifact-free results (coughing, delayed onset, etc.); (3) sustained expiration for at least 3 s; (4) three readings within 10% of largest effort; and (5) satisfactory performance as observed by the tester.

Reference

Lemen RJ. Pulmonary function testing in the office, clinic, and home. In Chernick V, Kendig EL Jr, eds. *Kendig's Disorders of the Respiratory Tract in Children*, 5th edn. Philadelphia, PA: WB Saunders, 1990:147–53

BREATHING INDEX

Use

To predict successful weaning from mechanical ventilation.

Formula

$$BI = \frac{f}{V_t}$$

BI = breathing index
f   = breaths per minute (spontaneous)
V_t = tidal volume (spontaneous)

Interpretation

A BI of less than 100 is predictive of successful weaning from a ventilator in adults. This single index has shown high sensitivity and specificity in adults, but data in pediatric patients are not available. Other traditional indices have also not been reliable in children.

References

Kacmarek R, Custer JR, Fugate JH. Mechanical ventilation. In Todres ID, Fugate JH, eds. *Critical Care in Infants and Children*, 1st edn. Boston, MA: Little Brown, 1996:175

McWilliams B. Mechanical ventilation in pediatric patients. In Hilman BC, ed. *Pediatric Respiratory Disease: Diagnosis and Treatment*. Philadelphia, PA: WB Saunders, 1993:909–10

Schultz TR, Lin RJ, Watzman HM, *et al*. Weaning children from mechanical ventilation: a prospective randomized trial of protocol-directed versus physician-directed weaning. *Respir Care* 2001;46:772–82

Yang K, Tobin MJ. A prospective study of indexes predicting outcomes of trials of weaning from mechanical ventilation. *N Engl J Med* 1991;324:1445–50

EFFECTIVE STATIC COMPLIANCE

Use

To provide information on the mechanics of the respiratory system in patients receiving mechanical ventilation.

Formula

$$C_{ES} = \frac{V_{ET}}{P_{plat} - PEEP}$$

$$C_{ES} = \text{effective static compliance (ml/cmH}_2\text{O)}$$
$$V_{ET} = \text{expired mechanical tidal volume (ml)}$$
$$P_{plat} = \text{plateau pressure (cmH}_2\text{O)}$$
PEEP = positive end-expiratory pressure plus auto-PEEP if present (cmH$_2$O)

Interpretation

In large adolescents compliance may reach normal adult levels of 70–100 ml/cmH$_2$O. Small pediatric patients may have a normal compliance of 3–4 ml/cmH$_2$O. Single values of C_{ES} have limited usefulness. Decreasing values indicate the lung–thoracic system is stiffer, as in worsening pneumothorax, pneumonia and pulmonary edema. Increasing values indicate a less stiff system or improving conditions.

Reference

Kacmarek R, Custer JR, Fugate JH. Mechanical ventilation. In Todres ID, Fugate JH, eds. *Critical Care in Infants and Children*, 1st edn. Boston, MA: Little Brown, 1996:164–5

AIRLINE TRAVEL

Use

To estimate the tolerance to airline travel of patients with impaired oxygenation due to airflow obstruction. Airliners are cabin pressurized to the height equivalent of between 6000 and 8000 feet.

Formula 1

$$PaO_{2Alt} = 22.8 - (2.74 \times Alt) + (0.68 \times PaO_{2SL})$$

Formula 2

$$PaO_{2Alt} = (0.45 \times PaO_{2SL}) + (0.38 \times FEV_1) + 2.44$$

Formula 3

$$PaO_{2Alt} = 17.802 + (0.417 \times PaO_{2SL})$$

PaO_{2Alt} = arterial oxygen tension at altitude (mmHg)
Alt = cabin pressurized altitude (feet/1000)
PaO_{2SL} = arterial oxygen tension at sea level (mmHg)
FEV_1 = patient's forced expiratory volume in 1 s (percent of predicted)

81

Interpretation

All studies have been done in adults, mostly the elderly. In those adult normocapneic patients, a PaO_{2Alt} of > 50 mmHg have not required supplemental oxygen. This translates to a PaO_2 of > 68 mmHg at sea level for those flying at 8000 feet cabin altitude. The majority of young patients who have PaO_2 greater than 55 mmHg can tolerate cabin altitudes of 8000 feet equivalent. With a PaO_2 of 55 mmHg at sea level, the PaO_{2Alt} at 8000 feet would be near 40 mmHg, and arterial hemoglobin oxygen saturation still 75%. Apparently an increase in heart rate and minute ventilation can still provide adequate oxygen delivery. This is also facilitated by the better oxygen release on the steep part of the oxyhemoglobin dissociation curve.

References

Desmond KJ, Coates AL, Beaudry PH. Relationship between partial pressure of arterial oxygen and airflow limitation in children with cystic fibrosis. *Can Med Assoc J* 1984;131:325–6

Dillard TA, Berg BW, Rajagopal KR, *et al*. Hypoxemia during air travel in patients with chronic obstructive pulmonary disease. *Ann Intern Med* 1989;111:362–7

Dillard TA, Moores LK, Bilello KL, Phillips YY. The preflight evaluation: a comparison of the hypoxia inhalation test with hypobaric exposure. *Chest* 1995;107:352–7

Gold WM. Pulmonary function testing. In Murray JF, Nadel JA, eds. *Textbook of Respiratory Medicine*, 2nd edn. Philadelphia, PA: WB Saunders, 1989:880

Gong H, Tashkin DP, Lee EY, Simmons MS. Hypoxia–altitude simulation test; evaluation of patients with chronic airway obstruction. *Am Rev Resp Dis* 1994;130: 980–6

Kurland G. Adaptation to high altitude. In Hilman B, ed. *Pediatric Respiratory Disease: Diagnosis and Treatment*. Philadelphia, PA: WB Saunders, 1993:414–15

Wall MA, LaGesse PC. Breathing in unusual environments. In Taussig LM, Landau LI, eds. *Pediatric Respiratory Medicine*. St Louis, MO: Mosby, 1999:130–3

ENDOTRACHEAL TUBE SIZE

Use

To estimate the endotracheal tube size for pediatric patients.

Formula 1 – internal diameter

$$D_i = \frac{A}{4} + 4$$

D_i = internal diameter (mm)
A = age (years)

Interpretation

The formula is useful from 1 to 16 years. Prematures require 2.5–3.0 mm, newborns 3.0–3.5 mm, and 6-month-old infants 3.5 mm. After insertion, there should be an air leak (no greater than 25 cmH$_2$O pressure) to avoid trauma to the larynx and trachea.

Formula 2 – oral tracheal tube depth of intubation

$$L_o = \frac{A}{2} + 13$$

Alternative formula: $L_o = A + 10$

L_o = length of oral tube (cm)
A = age (years)

Interpretation

The formula is useful from 1 to 16 years. Prematures require 8 cm, newborns 9 cm and 6-month-old infants 10 cm. Measurement is from the lips.

Formula 3 – nasotracheal tube depth of intubation

$$L_n = \frac{A}{2} + 16$$

L_n = length of nasal tube (cm)
A = age (years)

Interpretation

The formula is useful from 1 to 16 years. Prematures require 11 cm, newborns 12 cm and 6-month-old infants 14 cm. Measurement is from the external nares.

Reference

Wood RE. Diagnostic and therapeutic procedures in pediatric pulmonary patients. In Taussig LM, Landau LI, eds. *Pediatric Respiratory Medicine*. St Louis, MO: Mosby, 1999:251

RENAL FUNCTION

CREATININE CLEARANCE

Use

To estimate glomerular filtration rate.

Formula

$$Cl_{Cr} = \frac{Cr_u \times V}{Cr_p} \times \frac{1.73}{BSA}$$

Cl_{Cr} = creatinine clearance (ml/min/1.73 m^2)
Cr_u = urine creatinine (mg/24 h)
V = volume of urine in 24 h (ml)
Cr_p = plasma creatinine (mg/dl)
BSA = body surface area (m^2)

Interpretation

The Cl_{Cr} actually measures the theoretical volume of plasma cleared of creatinine in a finite period of time (ml/min). While creatinine clearance is used to estimate glomerular filtration rate (GFR), it usually overestimates GFR because some creatinine is secreted by the renal tubules. GFR (and therefore Cl_{Cr}) also varies with age in infants below 2 years, even after correction for surface area. Additionally, Cl_{Cr} is notoriously inaccurate in children for a variety of reasons. Accurately timed urine collections are difficult in infants and children, and non-creatinine chromagens interfere with creatinine measurement in the laboratory.

Range of normal values for Cl_{Cr} (and GFR) are as follows:

Age	Range (ml/min/1.73 m²)
Premature	
(< 34 weeks' gestation)	
2–8 days	11–15
4–28 days	15–28
30–90 days	40–65
Term neonates	
(> 34 weeks' gestation)	
2–8 days	17–60
4–28 days	26–68
30–90 days	30–86
1–6 months	39–114
6–12 months	49–157
12–19 months	62–191
2–12 years	89–165

References

Heilbron WE, Holliday MA, Al-Dahwi A, Kogan BA. Expressing glomerular filtration rate in children. *Pediatr Nephrol* 1991;5:5–11

Wong AF, Bounger AM, Gambertoglio JG. Pharmacokinetics and drug dosing in children with decreased renal function. In Holliday MA, Barratt TM, Avner ED, eds. *Pediatric Nephrology*, 3rd edn. Baltimore, MD: Williams & Wilkins, 1994:1305–6

CREATININE CLEARANCE ESTIMATE

Use

To estimate creatinine clearance without the need for urine collection. Creatinine clearance is used clinically as a substitute for actually measuring glomerular filtration rate (GFR).

Formula

$$Cl_{Cr} = \frac{k \times L}{P_{Cr}}$$

$$
\begin{aligned}
Cl_{Cr} &= \text{creatinine clearance (ml/min/1.73 m}^2) \\
k &= \text{constant (see table)} \\
L &= \text{body length (cm)} \\
P_{Cr} &= \text{plasma creatinine concentration (mg/dl)}
\end{aligned}
$$

k values vary with body size and sex

Age	k value
Preterm	0.33
Full term	0.45
Children and adolescent girls	0.55
Adolescent boys	0.70

Interpretation

Range of normal values for Cl_{Cr} (and GFR) are as follows:

Age	Range (ml/min/1.73 m²)
Premature	
(< 34 weeks' gestation)	
2–8 days	11–15
4–28 days	15–28
30–90 days	40–65
Term neonates	
(> 34 weeks' gestation)	
2 8 days	17–60
4–28 days	26–68
30–90 days	30–86
1–6 months	39–114
6–12 months	49–157
12–19 months	62–191
2 years to adult	89–165

References

Schwartz GJ, Brion LP, Spitzer A. The use of plasma creatinine concentration for estimating glomerular filtration rate in infants, children and adolescents. *Pediatr Clin North Am* 1987;34:571–90

Schwartz GJ, Gauthier B. A simple estimate of glomerular filtration rate in adolescent boys. *J Pediatr* 1985;106:522–6

Wong AF, Bounger AM, Gambertoglio JG. Pharmacokinetics and drug dosing in children with decreased renal function. In Holliday MA, Barratt TM, Avner ED, eds. *Pediatric Nephrology*, 3rd edn. Baltimore, MD: Williams & Wilkins, 1994:1305–6

CREATININE CLEARANCE ESTIMATE IN SMALL INFANTS

Use

To estimate creatinine clearance without the need for urine collection in small infants. Creatinine clearance is used as a substitute for actually measuring glomerular filtration rate (GFR). This estimation of GFR or creatinine clearance is especially useful clinically for drug dose alteration in small infants with renal functional impairment.

Formula

$$Cl_{Cr} = 120 \times (Wt/70)^{0.73} \times (0.4/S_{Cr}) \times MF$$

Cl_{Cr} = creatinine clearance (ml/min)
Wt = weight (kg)
S_{Cr} = serum creatinine (mg/dl)
MF = maturation factor (see table)

The above formula is valid in infants preterm to 1 year post-conception.

Age	Maturation factor
< 36 weeks post-conception and ≤ 10 days postnatal	0.18
< 36 weeks post-conception and > 10 days postnatal	0.36
≥ 36 weeks post-conception and ≤ 10 days postnatal	0.25
≥ 36 weeks post-conception and > 10 days postnatal	0.50
> 44 weeks post-conception (max 52 weeks or 12 months)	0.50 + (age in months/24)

Interpretation

The formula is an estimate of raw GFR (in ml/min) and must be converted to a corrected clearance by multiplying the raw value by surface area/1.73 m^2 to compare with normal tables, as shown in the table below. Range of normal values for Cl_{Cr} (and GFR) in ml/min/1.73 m^2 are as follows:

Age	Range (ml/min/1.73 m^2)
Premature	
(< 34 weeks' gestation)	
2–8 days	11–15
4–28 days	15–28
30–90 days	40–65
Term neonates	
(> 34 weeks' gestation)	
2–8 days	17–60
4–28 days	26–68
30–90 days	30–86
1–6 months	39–114
6–12 months	49–157
12–19 months	62–191
2 years to adult	89–165

Reference

Wong AF, Bounger AM, Gambertoglio JG. Pharmacokinetics and drug dosing in children with decreased renal function. In Holliday MA, Barratt TM, Avner ED, eds. *Pediatric Nephrology*, 3rd edn. Baltimore, MD: Williams & Wilkins, 1994:1306

PERCENT OF NORMAL GLOMERULAR FILTRATION RATE

Use

To estimate percent of normal glomerular filtration rate (GFR) using creatinine clearance as a function of GFR. Creatinine clearance is used as a substitute for actually measuring GFR. An estimation of percent of normal GFR is especially useful clinically for drug dose alteration in small infants and patients with renal functional impairment.

Formula

$$\%Cl_{Cr_n} = \frac{Cl_{Cr_a}}{Cl_{Cr_n}} \times 100$$

Cl_{Cr_n} = normal creatinine clearance for age
Cl_{Cr_a} = actual creatinine clearance

Note: The units for creatinine clearance are either ml/min or ml/min/1.73 m^2. In determining the percent of normal, it is imperative that the methodology of measuring or estimating both actual and normal clearance is the same, and that both measurements are either corrected or uncorrected for surface area. (See 'estimates of creatinine clearance' above)

Interpretation

Dosage regimens will frequently indicate dosage based on renal function (i.e. GFR). Tables frequently indicate dosage recommendation for 50–100% GFR, 10–50% GFR, < 10% GFR and those with 0% GFR (dialysis patients).

Age	Serum creatinine (mg/dl)
Premature	
(< 34 weeks' gestation)	
< 2 weeks old	0.9
≥ 2 weeks old	0.8
Term neonates	
(> 34 weeks' gestation)	
< 2 weeks old	0.5
≥ 2 weeks old	0.4
2 weeks to 1 year	0.4

This table can be used to derive normal creatinine clearance from serum creatinine in infants under 1 year.

The following formulas provide an estimation of normal serum creatinine in children and young adults aged 1–20 years.

Boys:

$$S_{Cr} = 0.35 + 0.025A$$

Girls:

$$S_{Cr} = 0.35 + 0.018A$$

A = age (years)

References

Wong AF, Bounger AM, Gambertoglio JG. Pharmacokinetics and drug dosing in children with decreased renal function. In Holliday MA, Barratt TM, Avner ED, eds. *Pediatric Nephrology*, 3rd edn. Baltimore, MD: Williams & Wilkins, 1994:1305–11

Yared A, Ichikawa I. Renal blood flow and glomerular filtration rate. In Holliday MA, Barratt TM, Avner ED, eds. *Pediatric Nephrology*, 3rd edn. Baltimore, MD: Williams & Wilkins, 1994:74

URINE PROTEIN/CREATININE RATIO

Use

To determine whether proteinuria is sufficiently high to pursue a quantitative 24-h urine collection.

Formula

$$\text{Ratio} = \frac{U_{pr}}{U_{Cr}}$$

U_{pr} = urine protein (mg/dl)
U_{Cr} = urine creatinine (mg/dl)

Interpretation

Significant proteinuria is indicated by a ratio of > 0.2 (> 0.5 in small infants). A ratio of > 1.0 indicates nephrotic-range proteinuria.

References

Roy S III. Hematuria. *Pediatr Ann* 1996;2:284

Roy S III. Hematuria. *Pediatr Rev* 1998;19:211

TRANSTUBULAR POTASSIUM CONCENTRATION GRADIENT

Use

To identify whether hyperkalemia is secondary to mineralocorticoid deficiency (or unresponsiveness).

Formula

$$TTKG = \frac{K_u}{K_s} \times \frac{S_{OSM}}{U_{OSM}}$$

TTKG	=	transtubular potassium gradient
K_U	=	urine potassium (mEq/l)
K_s	=	serum potassium (mEq/l)
U_{OSM}	=	urine osmolality (mOsm/kg)
S_{OSM}	=	serum osmolality (mOsm/kg)

Interpretation

This formula is helpful in patients with some degree of renal insufficiency when fractional potassium excretion should be increased. If the hyperkalemia is associated with a mineralocorticoid deficiency or unresponsiveness, the TTKG will be low. Mean gradient for normal children is 6.0 (range 4.1–10.5), and for normal infants 7.8 (range 4.9–15.5). Any values below these limits can be interpreted as indicating mineralocorticoid deficiency or unresponsiveness.

Urinary potassium concentration, and the urine/serum potassium ratio, are difficult to interpret, since they do not account for the variability in urine potassium concentration as a function of water reabsorption in the collecting duct. Also, fractional potassium excretion is not of much clinical utility, since potassium is primarily secreted and not dependent on filtration.

References

Restigar A, DeFronzo RA. Clinical disorders of fluid, electrolyte, and acid–base. In Schrier RW, Gottschalk CW, eds. *Diseases of the Kidney*, 5th edn. Boston, MA: Little Brown, 1993:2658–9

West ML, Mardsen PA, Richardson RMA, *et al*. New clinical approach to evaluate disorders of potassium excretion. *Miner Electrolyte Metab* 1985;12:234–8

URINARY PROTEIN SELECTIVITY RATIO

Use

To determine the excretion of high molecular protein relative to albumin in patients with heavy proteinuria.

Formula

$$\text{Ratio} = \frac{U_{IgG} \times P_A}{P_{IgG} \times U_A}$$

$$
\begin{aligned}
U_{IgG} &= \text{urine IgG concentration (g/dl)} \\
P_{IgG} &= \text{plasma IgG concentration (g/dl)} \\
P_A &= \text{plasma albumin concentration (g/dl)} \\
U_A &= \text{urine albumin concentration (g/dl)}
\end{aligned}
$$

Interpretation

In patients with heavy proteinuria (nephrotic range), a selectivity ratio of < 0.1 predicts steroid responsiveness, and a ratio of > 0.2 steroid resistance.

Reference

Barratt TM, Macaulay D. Renal disease in childhood. In Black DAK, ed. *Renal Disease*, 3rd edn. Oxford: Blackwell Scientific Publications, 1972:805

URINARY ALBUMIN/CREATININE RATIO

Use

To identify microalbuminuria in patients with diabetes mellitus as an indicator of renal disease.

Formula

$$\text{Ratio} = \frac{Alb_u}{Cr_u}$$

$$
\begin{aligned}
Alb_u &= \text{urine albumin (mg)} \\
Cr_u &= \text{urine creatinine (g)}
\end{aligned}
$$

Interpretation

Normal ratio is 1.24–10.34. Significant albuminuria is present when the ratio exceeds 30. (This is equivalent to 3.5 mg/mmol of creatinine.) Microalbuminuria is considered present in adults when urinary excretion rate is 20–200 µg/min, but in children this excretion rate will vary with body size. The ratio obviates the need for 24-h urine collections, since creatinine excretion is proportional to body size. There is a 40% day-to-day variation in albumin excretion, and there may be up to 25% greater excretion during the day than during the night. The first voided urine specimen should be used for determining the ratio.

The urine albumin/creatinine ratio is useful in diagnosing early diabetic nephropathy, which rarely occurs until diabetes is present for more than 5 years.

References

Dalton RN, Haycock GB. Laboratory investigation. In Holliday MA, Barratt TM, Avner ED, eds. *Pediatric Nephrology*, 3rd edn. Baltimore, MD: Williams & Wilkins, 1994:402–3

Fioretto P, Morgensen CE, Mauer SM. Diabetic nephropathy. In Holliday MA, Barratt TM, Avner ED, eds. *Pediatric Nephrology*, 3rd edn. Baltimore, MD: Williams & Wilkins, 1994:578

Gatling W, Knight C, Hill RD. Screening for early diabetic nephropathy. Which sample to detect microalbuminuria. *Diabetic Med* 1985;2:451–5

FRACTIONAL EXCRETION OF SODIUM

Use

To distinguish between pre-renal azotemia and acute renal failure.

Formula

$$FE_{Na} = \frac{U_{Na} \times P_{Cr}}{U_{Cr} \times P_{Na}} \times 100$$

FE_{Na} = fractional excretion of sodium (%)
U_{Na} = urine sodium concentration (mg/dl)
P_{Cr} = plasma creatinine concentration (mg/dl)
U_{Cr} = urine creatinine concentration (mg/dl)
P_{Na} = plasma sodium concentration (mg/dl)

Interpretation

Normal fractional sodium excretion is 0.01–10% and under normal circumstances is a reflection of sodium intake. Under conditions of hypovolemia (as in dehydration), FE_{Na} is generally under 1%. The measurement of FE_{Na} is helpful in oliguric states, distinguishing hypovolemia (pre-renal azotemia) from acute renal failure. FE_{Na} is less than 1% in pre-renal azotemia, and greater than 1% in acute renal failure. However, in prematures and newborns, FE_{Na} may be as high as 2.5% in pre-renal azotemia.

A spot urine is satisfactory for measuring FE_{Na}, but all measurements must be made on the same urine sample, and the blood studies must be made at the time of urine collection. Diuretic therapy will make this measurement invalid.

References

Cogan MG. *Fluid and Electrolyte Physiology and Pathophysiology.* Norwalk, CT: Appleton & Lange, 1991:38

Dalton NR, Haycock GB. Laboratory investigation. In Holliday MA, Barratt TM, Avner ED, eds. *Pediatric Nephrology*, 3rd edn. Baltimore, MD: Williams & Wilkins, 1994:397–8

Mathew OP. Neonatal renal failure: usefulness of diagnostic indices. *Pediatrics* 1980;65:57–60

CREATININE INDEX

Use

To provide an estimate of the expected 24-h urine creatinine excretion based on body weight. The estimate can be used to assess the accuracy of a 24-h urine collection. Urine collection is a major source of error in creatinine clearance measurement.

Formula

$$Cr_i = \frac{Cr_e}{Wt}$$

Cr_i = creatinine index (mg/kg/day)
Cr_e = creatinine excretion (mg/24 h)
Wt = body weight (kg)

Interpretation

The creatinine index is in the range of 15–20 mg/kg/day in boys, and 10–15 mg/kg/day in girls and infants. For adult men the index is 20–26 mg/kg/day, for adult women 14–22 mg/kg/day. These values are lower with decreased muscle mass.

In preterm infants in the first 2 weeks of life, creatinine excretion correlates with birth weight, body length and gestational age, but the strongest correlation is with birth weight according to the following equation:

Formula (preterm first 2 weeks)

$$Cr_i = 9.4 \times (BW - 1.48)$$

Cr_i = creatinine index (mg/kg/day)
BW = birth weight (kg)

References

Cogan MG. *Fluid and Electrolyte Physiology and Pathophysiology.* Norwalk, CT: Appleton & Lange, 1991:20

Sutphen JL. Anthropometric determinants of creatinine excretion in preterm infants. *Pediatrics* 1982;69:719–23

Yared A, Ichikawa I. Renal blood flow and glomerular filtration rate. In Holliday MA, Barratt TM, Avner ED, eds. *Pediatric Nephrology*, 3rd edn. Baltimore, MD: Williams & Wilkins, 1994:73–4

URINE CALCIUM/CREATININE RATIO

Use

To determine whether urinary calcium excretion is abnormally high, i.e. whether hypercalciuria exists.

Formula

$$R - \frac{U_{Ca}}{U_{Cr}}$$

R = ratio
U_{Ca} = urine calcium concentration (mg/dl)
U_{Cr} = urine creatinine concentration (mg/dl)

Interpretation

Hypercalciuria is considered present if the ratio is above the 95th centile for age. Patients with high ratios are at risk for urinary calcium stone formation.

Age	95th centile for Ca/Cr ratio (mg/mg)
5 days to 7 months	0.86
7–18 months	0.60
19 months to 6 years	0.42
over 6 years	0.22

Reference

Sargent JD, Stukel TA, Kresel J, Klein RZ. Normal values for random urinary calcium to creatinine ratios in infancy. *J Pediatr* 1993;123:393–7

URINE OSMOLALITY/PLASMA OSMOLALITY RATIO IN OLIGURIA

Use

To determine the cause of oliguria (usually urine volume below 300 ml/m^2 or below one-fifth maintenance fluid requirement).

Formula

$$R = \frac{U_{OSM}}{P_{OSM}}$$

R	=	ratio
U_{OSM}	=	urine osmolality (mOsm/kg H_2O)
P_{OSM}	=	plasma osmolality (mOsm/kg H_2O)

Interpretation

A ratio greater than 1.3 in the presence of oliguria suggests a prerenal cause (renal hypoperfusion). A ratio less than 1.3 suggests renal failure. A value greater than 2.0, in the presence of high urine sodium concentration (> 40 mEq/l) is seen in syndromes of inappropriate anti-diuretic hormone (SIADH).

While the U_{OSM}/P_{OSM} ratio is helpful clinically, the use of additional parameters can better identify the cause of oliguria, as shown in the following table (parentheses indicate neonate):

Parameter	Pre-renal	Renal failure	SIADH
U_{OSM}/P_{OSM} ratio	> 1.3	< 1.3	> 2.0
Urine specific gravity	≥ 1.020 (≥ 1.015)	< 1.010 (< 1.015)	> 1.020
Urine Na (mEq/l)	< 10 (< 20)	> 40 (> 40)	> 40
Urine osmolality (mOsm/kg H_2O)	> 500 (> 350)	< 350 (< 300)	> 500
Renal failure index*	< 1.0 (< 3.0)	> 1.0 (> 3.0)	> 1.0
Fractional excretion of Na (%)*	< 1.0 (< 2.5)	> 1.0 (> 3.0)	≈ 1.0

* Described on page 92

References

Rogers MC. *Textbook of Pediatric Intensive Care*. Baltimore, MD: Williams & Wilkins, 1992

Siegel NJ, Van Why SK, Boydstun II, *et al*. Acute renal failure. In Holliday MA, Barratt TM, Avner ED, eds. *Pediatric Nephrology*, 3rd edn. Baltimore, MD: Williams & Wilkins, 1994:1187

RENAL FAILURE INDEX

Use

To distinguish between pre-renal azotemia and acute renal failure.

Formula

$$RFI = \frac{U_{Na}}{U_{Cr}/P_{Cr}}$$

RFI	=	renal failure index
U_{Na}	=	urine sodium concentration (mg/dl)
U_{Cr}	=	urine creatinine concentration (mg/dl)
P_{Cr}	=	plasma creatinine concentration (mg/dl)

Interpretation

The renal failure index is an alternative to the fractional sodium excretion. Under conditions of hypovolemia (as in dehydration), RFI is generally less than 1.0. As with the FE_{Na}, this measurement is helpful in oliguric states, distinguishing hypovolemia (pre-renal azotemia) from acute renal failure. RFI is less than 1.0 in pre-renal azotemia, and greater than 1.0 in acute renal failure. However, in prematures and newborns, RFI may be as high as 3.0 in pre-renal azotemia.

A spot urine is satisfactory for measuring RFI, but all measurements must be made on the same urine sample, and the serum sodium drawn at the time of urine collection. Diuretic therapy will make this measurement invalid.

References

Rogers MC. *Textbook of Pediatric Intensive Care*. Baltimore, MD: Williams & Wilkins, 1992

Saxton CR, Seldin DW. Clinical interpretation of laboratory values. In Kokko JP, Tannen RL, eds. *Fluid and Electrolytes*. Philadelphia, PA: WB Saunders, 1986:51

STATISTICS

SENSITIVITY, SPECIFICITY AND PREDICTIVE VALUES

Use

To evaluate the accuracy and utility of any determinant such as a laboratory test, physical sign, historical data, etc. in diagnosis.

True-positive, false-positive, false-negative and true-negative test results

	Disease	
Test	*Present*	*Absent*
Positive	A* (true positive)	B* (false positive)
Negative	C* (false negative)	D* (true negative)

* A, B, C, D are numbers of persons.

Sensitivity (Se) (%)

Formula

$$Se = \frac{A}{A + C} \times 100$$

Sensitivity measures the percentage of those with the disease that will test positive.

Specificity (Sp) (%)

Formula

$$Sp = \frac{D}{D + B} \times 100$$

Specificity measures the percentage of those without the disease that will test negative.

Positive predictive value (PPV) (%)

Predictive value of a positive test.

Formula

$$PPV = \frac{A}{A + B} \times 100$$

Positive predictive value measures the percentage of those with a positive test that will have the disease. Contrast this with sensitivity, which is the percentage of those having the disease that will have a positive test.

Negative predictive value (NPV) (%)

Predictive value of a negative test.

Formula

$$NPV = \frac{D}{C + D} \times 100$$

Negative predictive value measures the percentage of those with a negative test that will be disease-free. Contrast this with specificity, which is the percentage of those without the disease who will have a negative test.

References

Bailar, JC III, Mostellar F. Medical technology assessment. In Bailar JC III, Mostellar F, eds. *Medical Use of Statistics*, 2nd edn. Boston: New England Journal of Medicine Books, 1992:393–411

Sackett DL, Hayes RB. Summarizing the effects of therapy: a new table and some more terms. *ACP Journal Club* 1997;127:A15–A16

Smith JE, Winkler RL, Fryback DG. The first positive: computing positive predictive value. *Ann Intern Med* 2000;132:804–9

Note: Each issue of *ACP Journal Club* contains a glossary of statistical terms commonly used in the medical literature.

RISK EVALUATION

Use

To indicate the strength of association between two factors, such as a disease and a treatment.

Number of persons with and without the disease in the presence and absence of a particular factor

Factor	Disease	No disease
Present	A*	B*
Absent	C*	D*

* A, B, C, D are numbers of persons.

Risk

Risk can be expressed as a fraction (such as 0.1) or a percentage (such as 10%). Risk is the rate or probability of a given outcome within a specific group. For example, we can speak of the disease risk for treated and control groups. A rate becomes a probability when known results are used to predict future results. Probability becomes risk when the positive outcome is undesirable.

Formulas

$$P_A = \frac{A}{A+B}$$

$$P_c = \frac{C}{C+D}$$

$$P_A = \text{rate in treated group}$$
$$P_c = \text{rate in control group}$$

Risk varies from 0 (no risk) to 1 (100% risk).

Relative risk (RR)

The relative risk is the ratio of the disease risk in the treated and in the control groups.

Formula

$$RR = \frac{P_A}{P_c}$$

$$= \frac{\left(\frac{A}{A+B}\right)}{\left(\frac{C}{C+D}\right)}$$

Interpretation

(1) RR < 1 suggests an effective therapy.
(2) RR > 1 suggests that the factor augments the disease.

Absolute risk reduction (ARR)

The absolute risk reduction is the difference in disease risk between the treated and control groups.

Formula

$$ARR = P_c - P_A$$

$$= \frac{C}{C+D} - \frac{A}{A+B}$$

Interpretation

A positive ARR indicates that the treatment is beneficial.

Relative risk reduction (RRR)

The RRR indicates the reduction of disease rate between the treated and control groups as compared to the disease rate in the control group. RRR = 1 − RR.

Formula

$$RRR = \frac{ARR}{P_c}$$

$$= 1 - \frac{\left(\frac{A}{A+B}\right)}{\left(\frac{C}{C+D}\right)}$$

Interpretation

RRR > 0 indicates an increasing degree of therapeutic effectiveness.
Risk evaluations are usually presented with a confidence interval (CI). For example, a 95% CI of 0.9–1.7 indicates that in 19 of 20 trials (95%) the result should fall between 0.9 and 1.7.

Odds

Odds compare within a group the number with the (undesirable) outcome with the number without that outcome. This is in contrast to risk, in which the number with the (undesirable) outcome is compared to the entire group, i.e. to the sum of those with and without the (undesirable) outcome.

Formulas

$$O_A = \frac{A}{B}$$

$$O_c = \frac{C}{D}$$

O_A = odds in treated group
O_C = odds in control group

Interpretation

Odds vary from 0 (no risk) to infinity (100% risk). Odds of 1 (i.e. 1 : 1 odds) correspond to a risk of 50%. This non-linear scale makes numerical values for odds more difficult to visualize than the comparable risk figures. When A and C are small, relative risk (RR) and odds ratio (OR) are approximately equal.

Odds Ratio (OR)

The odds ratio is the ratio of the disease odds in the treated and control groups.

Formula

$$OR = \frac{O_A}{O_C}$$

$$= \frac{\left(\frac{A}{B}\right)}{\left(\frac{C}{D}\right)}$$

Interpretation

OR < 1 indicates an effective therapy.

References

Havens PL. Evaluating medical literature: clinical epidemiology. In Behrman RE, Kliegman R, Nelson WE, Arvin AM, eds. *Nelson Textbook of Pediatrics*, 15th edn. Philadelphia: WB Saunders, 1995:6–7

Zelterman D, Louis TA. Contingency tables in medical studies. In Bailar JC III, Mostellar F, eds. *Medical Use of Statistics*, 2nd edn. Boston: New England Journal of Medicine Books, 1992:298

CONFIDENCE INTERVAL

Use

To quantify the reliability of a conclusion about an entire population drawn from a study sample of the population.

Formula

$$CI\ 95\% = (\bar{x} - 2se) \text{ to } (\bar{x} + 2se)$$

CI 95% = 95% confidence interval
$\bar{x}$ = mean (average) of the population sample
se = standard error

$$se = \frac{s}{\sqrt{n}}$$

s = standard deviation
n = size of population sample

$$s = \sqrt{\frac{\Sigma (x - \bar{x})^2}{n - 1}}$$

x	=	individual sample
$\Sigma (x - \bar{x})^2$	=	sum of the squares of the differences between each observation and the mean of the population.

Interpretation

Given a sample drawn from a population, the 95% confidence interval is a range surrounding its mean that contains, with 95% likelihood, the true mean of the entire population.

For example, if the average systolic blood pressure of a 10-year-old boy is 110, with a CI 95% of 90–130 then it is likely that the average systolic blood pressure of all comparable individuals is between 90 and 130.

In cases of risk and odds, if the confidence interval contains 1, then there is no evidence that the procedure or therapy significantly affected the outcome of the condition under study.

Reference

Rees DG. *Essential Statistics for Medical Practice*, 1st edn. London: Chapman and Hall, 1994:128–30

NUMBER NEEDED TO TREAT

Use

To quantify the impact of an intervention on an adverse outcome with particular reference to baseline (control) frequency of that outcome. Number needed to treat (NNT) is the average number of patients that must be treated for a disease before the treatment prevents that disease in one patient.

Number of persons with and without an adverse outcome in the presence and absence of treatment

Intervention	Adverse outcome	No adverse outcome
Present (treated)	A*	B*
Absent (control)	C*	D*

* A, B, C, D are numbers of persons.

Formula

$$NNT = \frac{1}{P_c - P_A}$$

$$= \frac{1}{\frac{c}{c+d} - \frac{a}{a+b}}$$

NNT	=	number needed to treat
P_c	=	rate in control group
P_A	=	rate in treated group

Interpretation

NNT compares the effectiveness of a prophylactic treatment to the relative rarity of the condition it is intended to treat. The NNT is the reciprocal of the ARR (page 99). It is intuitively apparent that the reduction by (for example) 25% of a frequent adverse outcome by treatment may be justified while the same percentage reduction of a rare adverse outcome may not be worth the cost of therapy and potential risk of side-effects.

The same formula can be used to calculate the number needed to harm (NNH) by interchanging the rate of an adverse effect with the treatment effect in the treatment and control groups. This then gives the number of patients treated to produce an adverse effect in one. Therapy may not be worth the cost and risk of side-effects if the NNH is small.

References

Chatellier G, Zapletal E, Lemaitre D, *et al*. The number needed to treat: a clinically useful nomogram in its proper context. *Br Med J* 1996;312:426–9 (Erratum *Br Med J* 1996;312:563)

Cook RJ, Sackett DL. The number needed to treat: a clinically useful measure of treatment effect. *Br Med J* 1995;310:452–4

Lubsen J, Hoes A, Grobbee D. Implications of trial results: the potentially misleading notions of number needed to treat and average duration of life gained. *Lancet* 2000;356:1757–9

APPENDICES

APPENDIX A

SI prefixes and measures

Prefix	Abbreviation	Factor	Linear measure	Volume measure
deci	d	10^{-1}	1 dm (decimeter) = 10^{-1} m	1 dl (deciliter) = 10^{-1} liter
centi	c	10^{-2}	1 cm (centimeter) = 10^{-2} m	1 cl (centiliter) = 10^{-2} l
milli	m	10^{-3}	1 mm (millimeter) = 10^{-3} m	1 ml (milliliter) = 10^{-3} l *
micro	μ	10^{-6}	1 μm (micrometer) = 10^{-6} m **	1 μl (microliter) = 10^{-6} l
nano	n	10^{-9}	1 nm (nanometer) = 10^{-9} m	1 nl (nanoliter) = 10^{-9} l
pico	p	10^{-12}	1 pm (picometer) = 10^{-12} m	1 pl (picoliter) = 10^{-12} l
femto	f	10^{-15}	1 fm (femtometer) = 10^{-15} m	1 fl (femtoliter) = 10^{-15} l

*, 1 ml = 1 cm^3 (almost exactly); **, the name 'micron' is deprecated but still used

APPENDIX B

Unit conversions

Class	Test	SI unit	Conventional unit
Chemistries	ALT, SGPT	1 µKat/l	58.82 U/l
	AST, SGOT	1 µKat/l	58.82 U/l
	Bilirubin	1 µmol/l	0.058 mg/dl
	BUN	1 mmol/l	2.80 mg/dl
	Calcium	1 mmol/l	4 mg/dl
	Carbon dioxide	1 mmol/l	1 mEq/l
	Chloride	1 mmol/l	1 mEq/l
	Cholesterol, total	1 mmol/l	38.61 mg/dl
	LDL	1 mmol/l	38.61 mg/dl
	HDL	1 mmol/l	38.61 mg/dl
	Creatinine	1 µmol/l	0.013 mg/dl
	Glucose	1 µmol/l	18.02 mg/dl
	Iron, total	1 µmol/l	5.59 mg/dl
	TIBC	1 mmol/l	5.59 mg/dl
	Lactate	1 mmol/l	9.01 mg/dl
	Magnesium	1 mmol/l	2.43 mg/dl
	Osmolality	1 mOsm/l	1 mmol/kg H_2O
	Phosphate	1 mmol/l	3.10 mg/dl
	Potassium	1 mmol/l	1 mEq/l
	Protein, total	1 g/l	0.1 g/dl
	Albumin	1 g/l	0.1 g/dl
	Globulin	1 g/l	0.1 g/dl
	Triglyceride	1 mmol/l	88.49 mg/dl
Endocrine	Follicle stimulating hormone (FSH)	1 U/ml	1 U/ml
	Insulin	1 pmol/l	0.144 µU/ml
	Luteinizing hormone (LH)	1 U/ml	1 U/ml
Hematology	Erythrocytes	10^{12}/l	10^6/mm^3 10^6/µl
	Erythrocyte indices		
	MCH	1 pg/cell	1 pg/cell
	MCHC	1 g/l	0.1 g/dl
	MCV	1 fl	1 µm^3
	Hemoglobin	1 g/l	0.1 g/dl
	Leukocytes	10^9/l	10^3/mm^3
	Platelets	10^9/l	10^3/µl

INDEX

fluids
  deficits 31–2
  extracellular (ECF) 15
  maintenance fluids 30–1
free water
  clearance 36
  deficit 34–5
  excess 32–3

gastrointestinal tract 48–9
glomerular filtration rate
  estimate 84–5
  percent of normal 88–9
glucose, serum 35, 45
glycolysis 63
growth *see* body metrics

Haycock formula 16
heart rate 21–3
height 18–19
hematocrit 50, 58
hemochromatosis 56
hemoglobin 12
  fetal 12, 13
  oxyhemoglobin dissociation curve
    13–14
hemoglobin C disease 54
hemolysis 38, 55
hemosiderosis 56
Henderson–Hasselbalch equation 1–2
hypercalcemia 24
  hypocalciuric 47
hyperchloremia, anion gap acidosis 10
hypercholesterolemia 62
hyperchromia 54
hyperglycemia 35–6, 64
  corrected serum sodium 35–6
hyperkalemia 24, 38
hypernatremia
  anion gap 10
  free water deficit 32, 34–5
hyperparathyroidism 46
hypertension 20, 25
  in prematures 25
hypoalbuminemia 39
hypocalciuria 94
hypocalciuric hypercalcemia 46, 47
hypochloremia 6
hypochromia 54

hypoglycemia 45, 64
hyponatremia 32–4
  dehydration 32, 33–4
  free water excess 32–3
hypoxemia 78

infectious disease 60–1
  catheter-related bacteremia 60
  cerebrospinal fluid/serum antibody
    index 60–1
insulin suppression test 45
intravenous drug infusion 75–6
iron deficiency 55, 56–7
iron poisoning 56
iron preparations 57
iron storage, transferrin saturation 55–6
ischemic heart disease 24

lactate/pyruvate ratio 63–4
lactic acidosis 63
lactose intolerance 49
lactulose 49
left ventricular shortening fraction 29
limb ratios 17–18
lipids, blood 62–3
liver 48–9
loading dose 74
luteinizing/follicle stimulating hormone
  ratio 46

maintenance fluids 30–1
metabolic acidosis 4–5
metabolic alkalosis 5–7
metabolic rate 66
metabolism 62–4
methanol 42–3
microalbuminuria 91
Mosteller's formula 16

negative predictive value (statistics) 98
nephrotic syndrome 48, 91
nesidioblastosis 45
nitrogen, protein 67
nitrogen balance 68–9
number needed to treat (statistics) 102–3
nutrition 65–73
  caloric expenditure 65–7
  dietary protein intake 70–1
  energy requirements 72–3